The Principles of
Homoeopathic
Philosophy

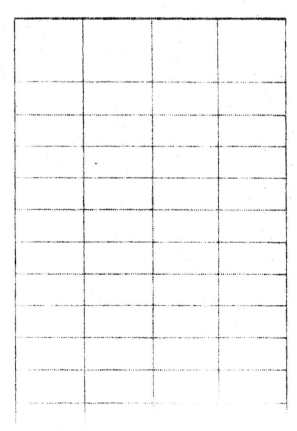

The Principles of
Homoeopathic
Philosophy

A self-directed learning text

Margaret Roy

Principal, The Scottish College of Homoeopathy and Practising Homoeopath

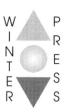

Winter Press
29 Horniman Drive
London SE23 3BJ

First published by Churchill Livingstone in 1994.
Published by Winter Press in 1999.

Text Copyright Margaret Roy 1999
Cover Copyright Winter Press 1999
Printed by Biddles of Guildford, Surrey

ISBN 1 874581 126

Contents

How to Use this Text

This distance-learning text aims to guide the student step-by-step through a learning programme on homoeopathic philosophy.

Each lesson contains instructive text with appropriate additional readings and a series of activities designed to develop a practical understanding of concepts, to widen the student's experience and to exercise practical skills.

You can use the text on your own, as an aid to the revision of existing knowledge of homoeopathic philosophy, or it can be used as a background text or to provide extra help in a professional training course.

Each student has his/her own approach. If some time has elapsed since your last period of serious study, Appendix I may prove useful. A good strategy might be to read the lesson, examine the readings given, then start the lesson again in earnest, doing the activities as they crop up, and finish by re-reading the set books or the summary of points noted from those and from this text. You should not worry if it is hard and does not all 'click' at first — learning is a challenge; there should be greater cause for concern if you find it easy! I have aimed in this text to provoke much thought and many questions, most of which should have been answered by the end of this course if I have been successful.

The text should begin to train the student to think homoeopathically. This involves using analytical skills and what may be a new perspective on the problem of disease. You will be encouraged to ask simple questions, even though these may appear superficial at first. The good student will be prepared to seek new insights into problems.

In addition, one of the best ways to study philosophy is in the Socratic fashion, which involves discussion among groups of open-minded people, sharing and challenging new concepts. Some of the exercises are best done in groups and in others, such as essays, the reader would benefit from the guidance of a tutor, even although the book is aimed at the individual. Beyond the level of this text, study should be increasingly practical, and should involve clinical training and personal tuition. In any event, I believe that this text will provide a useful introduction to classical homoeopathic medicine. May I wish you success in your studies.

Biggar, 1993   M.R.

Key to 'Activity' Symbols

The following symbol denotes an activity which involves . . .

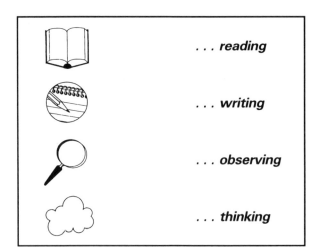

... reading

... writing

... observing

... thinking

An Introduction to Textbooks

Three books will be used alongside this text. The authors are masters of homoeopathy from different phases in its history. The language and concepts used are indicative of the period in which they practised and wrote. You will find them an interesting backdrop to your course.

Hahnemann Samuel, 1971, The Organon. B Jain, New Delhi

Kent J T 1970, Lectures on homoeopathic philosophy. B Jain, New Delhi

Vithoulkas G 1980, The Science of Homoeopathy. Thorsons, London

The Organon

The most important of these is of course Hahnemann's original masterpiece, *The Organon of the Rational Art of Healing*, first published in 1810 and translated from the original German by R.C. Dudgeon in 1893. Hahnemann put all his knowledge of the principles and philosophy of homoeopathy into this book. There are other translations, but the value of this edition is that the publishers have added footnotes comparing differences in the fifth edition of the *Organon* translated by Dudgeon, and the sixth edition translated by William Boericke. Dudgeon himself points out differences in the first five of Hahnemann's editions, and adds copious notes by way of explanation. One difficulty in using this text is that the English of 1893 is old-fashioned, and may prove heavy reading to some students. Some modern translations are not without error – in attitude if not meaning; it is important to go as close to the source as possible, so I have chosen this edition.

Within homoeopathy a controversy rages regarding the fifth and sixth editions of the *Organon*, and the repercussions of the differences between them. In Hahnemann's lifetime the sixth edition was not generally available, and indeed was not available till 1921, some time after his death. There are those who believe the sixth edition substantially changes the practice of homoeopathy, and thus we should pay careful attention to those parts where there is a difference. J.T. Kent did not have access to the sixth edition, and though his work is so influential within homoeopathy, it is suspected that the homoeopathy commonly known to us and called classical is really Kentian. The implication is that Hahnemann himself had already moved on!

Lectures in Homoeopathic Philosophy

J.T. Kent's understanding of homoeopathy is available in two main texts, *Lectures on Homoeopathic Philosophy* and *Lesser Writings*. The first of these, which will aid our study, was drawn together and published in 1900 from lectures delivered to postgraduate medical students studying homoeopathy. Much is a direct exposition of Hahnemann's *Organon* (fifth edition), but of course he adds many other pointers. His work is coloured by his adherence to Swedenborg's system of beliefs, but his approach is well tried in practice. In the USA, Kent was the most influential teacher and practitioner of homoeopathy during his lifetime, and this text will follow a mainly Kentian approach to homoeopathy.

The Science of Homoeopathy

George Vithoulkas' text *The Science of Homoeopathy* is the third textbook we will use. Vithoulkas' background as an engineer gives him a very practical approach to this subject, that takes away the vagueness and puts homoeopathic concepts into the terms of modern science with which we are more familiar today. Vithoulkas enables us to link our homoeopathic studies into our own field of experience, and also to make use of modern science's ideas of energy. In Hahnemann's day, concepts of energy were very rudimentary. It was Hahnemann's friend Lavoiser who first isolated oxygen and studied how it worked!

STUDY HINTS	Appropriate sections from these books will be given for reading and study after each lesson. It may be useful to read the portion of the text given both before and after studying the lesson, so as to enhance your understanding of the concepts studied.

LESSON ONE

Introduction to Homoeopathy

Headings: What is Homoeopathy?
Basic Homoeopathic Principles
The Homoeopathic Concept of Disease
Holistic and Natural Medicine
Medicine for the Individual

Aims: This lesson will summarize the whole course, giving an overall philosophy of homoeopathy into which the student can fit each subsequent lesson.

What is Homoeopathy?

The word homoeopathy derives from Greek root words meaning 'like cures like', i.e. that which causes disease can also cure it. This is a familiar concept, to be found in such terms as 'the hair of the dog that bit you': the hangover may indeed disappear with another drink, and the discomfort of the smoker is less so after another cigarette. The reasons are interesting. In homoeopathic experience it can be demonstrated that a medicine can cure high temperature and vomiting of yellow bile if that same medicine can cause those symptoms when taken by a healthy person.

This is very different from orthodox medicine which the homoeopath calls 'allopathy'. The method of cure in allopathy is to use medicine which creates the opposite effect in the body. Presented with a patient suffering from high temperature and vomiting bile, the allopath would be horrified to give a medicine that would cause these same symptoms. He or she would rather reach for a medicine that stops the vomiting (perhaps an antispasmodic that silences the relevant nerve) and lowers the temperature.

ACTIVITY 1

Several questions should be flowing through your mind already, such as, why doesn't homoeopathy make people more ill?

Take a little notebook and in it write down these questions and any others that may occur to you as you go through the text. If the text is challenging, many questions will arise as we go on, and I encourage you to question what is said. Homoeopathy is based on experience, and any sound system can stand up to very thorough investigation. Some exceptionally fine minds have investigated homoeopathy and found it thorough and scientific, so ponder on the questions. The answers will appear in the text as we go along.

Basic Homoeopathic Principles

There are five basic Laws of classical Homoeopathy:

The Law of Similars
The single remedy
The single dose
The minimum dose
The Law of Cure

I shall now go through a very simple explanation of these so you have an overview, and are therefore better able to understand the detail that follows in the other lessons.

The Law of Similars

It is from this fundamental tenet that homoeopathy derives its name. As Robert Davidson is so fond of quoting, 'it is not the remedy that is homoeopathic, but the reason for prescribing'.

Any therapeutic device may be homoeopathic if it is given on the understanding that it may initiate cure because *in other circumstances it may cause the same symptoms.*

One example of this might be to put one's finger under the hot tap after sustaining a burn rather than under the cold tap. Modern first aid directs us to put the finger under the cold tap, because the heat is dissipated and there is less damage to the part. This indeed makes sense, but try it under the hot tap! The burnt finger under the hot tap is more painful at first, but the pain goes sooner and the blister is much less likely to form.

To find out what it cures, each homoeopathic remedy has been given to healthy people until their health was disturbed and symptoms produced. This is called 'proving the remedy'. The symptoms produced in this way were then listed in detail as the symptom picture of the remedy. Since these are the symptoms the remedy can cause, these are the symptoms it can cure. The task of the homoeopath is therefore to elicit from the patient as many symptoms as possible, then to match the patient's symptom picture to that of a remedy. The closer the match, the more efficient the cure.

Homoeopathic remedies are not 'proven' (see Glossary) on sick people because their health is already disturbed. Similarly, animals are not used in homoeopathic provings as they are obviously unable to describe any symptoms they might have.

The symptoms pictures are listed in Materia Medicas, the most comprehensive of which is Allen's 12 volume Encyclopedia. In a Repertory, individual symptoms can be looked up as in a dictionary, to find all the remedies that have produced that particular symptom while testing. Kent's is the most commonly used Repertory.

ACTIVITY 2

You could explore this further by finding out the effects of arsenic poisoning, and then by looking up the homoeopathic Materia Medica to identify the symptoms that the remedy will cure.

The Single Remedy

What is termed classical homoeopathy treats the patient using only one remedy at a time. The reason for this is quite simple: when the remedies are tested they are tested singly, so that it can be argued that when the remedies are combined the effects are not known.

In France and Germany it is common for a patient to be given a group of remedies, perhaps as many as 12 in one treatment. The value of such treatment can be verified on the basis of clinical experience. In Britain, this is often called 'the Continental system'.

In this text we will study in depth the works of Hahnemann, Kent and Vithoulkas, who all see the single remedy as the only method of treatment.

The Single Dose

The concept of the single dose is based on the fact that the homoeopathic remedy does not cure the patient, nor is it designed to do so, but merely stimulates the body into action, because fundamentally the organism alone has the capacity to maintain health. When this self-correcting mechanism fails, how much energy does it need to get going again? Every homoeopath asks this question before giving a remedy, and on the basis of the answer will select the potency or strength of a remedy. Medicine is required only to create change. If change has already begun but is not yet visible, then it is possible to interfere and upset the healing process by giving another stimulus. So the homoeopath selects the amount of energy needed and gives it in one dose, then waits for results to assess the effect of the remedy.

Again this is advocated by Hahnemann, Kent and Vithoulkas, and it is the system we will look at in this book.

However it is also common practice to give multiple doses of homoeopathic remedies, usually in low potencies and often to chronically ill or older people. Antony Campbell in his book *The Two Faces of Homoeopathy* looks at this historical division among homoeopaths. Personally, I accept that both of these approaches may be correct in different circumstances. There are times when the vitality is weak and it needs a low energy stimulus repeated. It then becomes important to ask, how do you know the organism is reacting, and how is the organism reacting?

ACTIVITY 3 How many examples can you think of where too much repetition destroyed the effect you were trying to create?

The Minimum Dose

In the human organism the substances that create change and control the rate of change are present in minute amounts. These are the hormones and the enzymes. The role of the homoeopathic remedy is similar to that of enzymes and hormones in controlling the homoeostatic balance within the organism to maintain a functioning harmony between all parts. The homoeopathic remedy changes the organism, which then takes over. It is important to say the remedy *changes* the organism because, unlike in modern-day therapy, the remedy does not need to be present continually in order to create chemical changes. For example, the patient must continue to take diuretics, insulin, beta-blockers or anti-inflammatory drugs for rheumatism.

Hahnemann taught that additional doses of the medicine ceased to be therapeutic, and the body has to take out valuable time and energy to remove the excess medicine from the system. This delays cure.

ACTIVITY 4 What examples have you experienced first-hand that illustrate cure delayed by medicines in this way? This question will be easier for those already working with patients.

Potentization

Hahnemann went much further than the science of his day. He saw life as an energy he called the vital force, and he recognized that cure could be more effective if the medicine was also energized. He therefore developed the process he called potentization, because it made the medicine stronger.

STAGES OF POTENTIZATION

- A tincture is obtained of the medicine. The tincture of a plant may be obtained by boiling, soaking, drying and grinding it. Minerals are usually put into solution, or a tincture may be obtained of some metals by triturating them.
- The tincture of the remedy is diluted on a scale of 1:10 or 1:100. 1:10 is the decimal scale represented by an X or a D in Europe; 1:100 is the centesimal scale, represented by a C.

    The number that precedes the letter represents the number of times that the tincture has been diluted (1:10 or 1:100) and this represents the strength of the medicine. Hence Lachesis 6X has been diluted six times on the decimal scale and represents 6^{10} or 1 000 000. Lachesis 6C has been diluted six times on the centesimal scale, and represents 6^{100} or 1/1 000 000 000 000. 6C is thus much more potent than 6X (Fig. 1.1). The common potencies found in health stores are 6X and 6C. Other potencies used are 9X, 12X, 30X, 6C, 30C, 200C, 1M (a thousand), 10M – the C of the centesimal scale is most commonly omitted.
- Succussion occurs between each dilution. For years this was the more esoteric part of the process of potentization, involving vigorous shaking between each dilution stage. Traditionally, succussion involves thumping the medicine hard on the family bible! Nowadays a mechanical shaker is used, but there are many who profess that this is not adequate by comparison!

THE DYNAMIC LEVEL

To many, this method of remedy preparation smacks of charlatanism, and even today there are those critics of homoeopathy who say the medicine is so dilute that the only possible therapeutic effect is that of a placebo. However, Hahnemann claimed that this

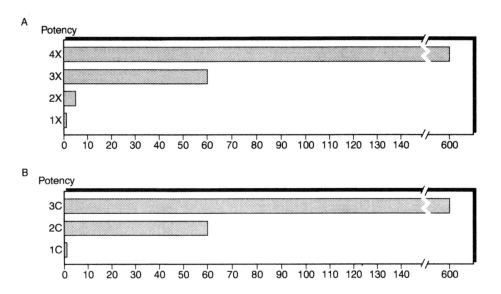

Fig. 1.1 A. Dilutions on the decimal scale. B. Dilutions on the centesimal scale.

method increased the potency of the remedy because it made it more 'dynamic'. The organism was not mere substance, the real active part was a force – the vital force – the nature of which was also 'dynamic', i.e. on the plane of causes.

Modern physics calls this dynamic force energy, and could explain how the vibratory structure of a substance may be changed by violently shaking it, as in succussion.

The Law of Cure

Although Hahnemann had a rudimentary idea of this, it was Constantine Hering who drew up the four laws that we know today.

To Hahnemann it was not enough to get rid of symptoms; patients had to be cured. Although he stated that cure was just the removal of those visible symptoms and nothing else was necessary or constituted cure, he later found out that patients might come back to him, perhaps 1 or 2 years later, and although the original symptoms were gone, other deeper more serious symptoms appeared, so that the reality of the patient's situation had become worse. Hering postulated that one did not need to wait so long, but could tell if cure was taking place by the change in the symptom picture. Symptoms should move very decidedly in specific directions if a cure is taking place.

FROM VITAL ORGANS TO LESS VITAL ORGANS

The most important direction is that symptoms should cease in vital organs, though frequently this may mean that symptoms appear or reappear in less vital organs, e.g. from the kidneys to the ear.

FROM WITHIN OUTWARDS

From internal organs symptoms should move outwards, e.g. symptoms disappear from mucus membranes lining the gut, and appear on the skin; thus also discharges of phlegm or diarrhoea could be a good sign.

FROM ABOVE DOWNWARDS

Symptoms should move from above downwards if on the way out, for example in skin problems, although more spots are visible these should be further down on a limb, or the trunk.

4

IN REVERSE ORDER OF APPEARANCE

The last symptoms to appear most often represent the deepening illness, so these will disappear first, and as the disease is cured the less serious early symptoms will return and then go. There is a distinct chronological order in this change of symptoms.

If all or any of these laws are present, then cure may be assumed to be taking place, as long as there are no contradictions. Of course, if the opposite is taking place, the patient may be deemed to be getting worse.

ACTIVITY 5

Let us look at an example of illness, preferably your own. How did the symptoms unfold?

In what order did the symptoms change as you proceeded to get better?

Find two to three examples of people with poor health. Question these people as to the kind of illnesses they have had in the past, and when. You should see less severe illness in the past and steadily more serious developments in health as time passes. Sometimes after early illnesses there will be a large gap of seemingly good health (really a lack of symptoms – compare the vitality at different periods) until suddenly a more serious illness appears.

The Homoeopathic Concept of Disease

Vitalism

Historically homoeopathy belongs to the school of medicine called vitalism, described further in Harris Coulter's *The Divided Legacy* and in Ortega's *Notes on the miasms*. Put simply, this means the homoeopath will never reduce the organism to a physical body of chemical or mechanical reactions. Instead, the homoeopath attempts to see the organism as a living form. Of course, such an attempt broaches many difficult philosophical questions which science has long since avoided by reducing life to chemical and mechanical answers, and so avoiding the big question of the mystery of life. The homoeopath, on the other hand, will talk of the vital force or principle, and will try to understand how the human organism works as a whole, and what kind of response it makes as a whole to its environment, or to ill health and disease.

In paragraphs 9 and 11 of the *Organon*, Hahnemann talks of an energy (dynamis) that gives life to the body, governing all bodily functions without exception, and creating a harmonious whole. The organism is able to keep itself healthy. It can correct homoeostatic balance, and repair tissues or direct energy where it is required. It is able to heal itself and if not, there must be something wrong with the coordinating process – the vital force.

Thus there is only **one possible disease** – the disturbance of the vital force: it is thrown into disharmony when its curative action is undermined.

What Happened to the Vital Force?

Lists of diseases mean nothing to the homoeopath. What he or she needs to find out is what happened to the vital force. What disturbed it? We cannot see the vital force, we can only observe the pattern of symptoms produced. To the homoeopath this is enough, because we already know that a medicine affects the health of a prover by creating waves of disturbance – symptoms. Thus using the Law of Similars we need only match the symptoms of the remedy to those produced by the disturbed vital force to bring about cure. How and why will be discussed later.

Symptoms Indicate Cure

One fundamental repercussion of this view of disease is that the homoeopath does not frown on symptoms as bad, but sees them as valuable indicators of the state of the vital force, and would even go further to say that the vital force produces symptoms in order to cure itself. Just as ripples are produced when we throw a stone into a pool, so symptoms are produced when we become ill; the ripples spread the energy of disturbance within the pool in exactly the same way that the symptoms dissipate the disturbance of the vital force. The symptoms are the process of cure, and thus it is important to understand their role, and to use them to identify the state of the organism. To create the most effective cure, we must learn to work with the body's own healing mechanisms and not use valuable energy forcing reactions that may not be appropriate.

ACTIVITY 6   Write down notes on your concept of health.
What goals is the homoeopath aiming at?
What expectations should each individual have as regards health?

Holistic and Natural Medicine

Before leaving this introduction a few words on topical terms will be appropriate.

Holistic Medicine

What do you understand by this term? It is usually understood to mean the treatment of the patient as a whole, taking into account his or her mental and emotional circumstances and environment. Each diseased part is seen in relation to the whole, to gain its proper significance.

This is very well developed in homoeopathy, where disease means that life itself is impaired or disturbed. Underlying the assessments of each homoeopathic case are such questions as:

• What is happening to the vital force (to the overall harmonious balance)?
• What has so disturbed this person as a whole that the vital force has had to produce this group of symptoms to overcome it?

Frequently the homoeopath is like Sherlock Holmes, searching for the point of change or cause of the original disturbance, which so disturbed the balance of the organism that drastic action was needed to avoid damage. Thus the patient may have symptoms a doctor would label bronchitis, but if these were believed to be caused by shock or grief, then the homoeopath would treat the shock or grief, and in so doing expect the bronchitis to remit spontaneously.

Another example may be boils that appear time and again in specific areas of the body. There are various ways of treating boils, with poultices etc., but a holistic method might look at the imbalance of the body's economy that enabled such a build up of debris. Treatment is from within to re-establish a sound economy, and this may well involve medication, exercise and diet.

Natural Medicine

Naturalistic treatment is often an abused term, merely referring to medicines used in their natural or unprocessed state. It is often applied in this way to homoeopathy, but from what we already known this is a misnomer, as all homoeopathic medicines are potentized, a process that could not really be described as natural. A more fundamental meaning of this term does, however, apply.

No-one knows the mechanism by which the organism creates or maintains health – it is a mystery of life. Homoeopathy is truly naturalistic because it does not interfere with the organism. Through observation, patterns in the change of the symptom picture have been noted. Once the path of disturbance is known, the homoeopath can give a medicine which initiates the process of cure by further stimulation of the organism along the same pattern of outward movement that it had already chosen for itself. The homoeopathic medicine is in such a small dose that it does not continue its action once the body has started to heal itself.

A homoeopathic medicine can also be used to speed up the process of cure by enhancing those very symptoms that the organism is using to expel the disease. This procedure recognizes the natural direction of cure and works within it, instead of imposing from without.

Medicine for the Individual

Today's patient wants natural holistic treatment, but also wants to know that his or her own peculiarities are dealt with. There is a profound fear at the root of this, and a mistrust that he or she will go on a conveyor belt and be out of his or her own control. There is no fear of this with homoeopathy, because so much information is needed in order to get the best fit of remedy to the patient's symptom picture.

There are no statistical averages in proving homoeopathic remedies. In fact, the exact opposite is the case because each remedy has to be distinguished clearly, and so in proving the remedy the homoeopath looks for those symptoms which are the strangest and most unique. When the patient's symptom picture is taken, the search is again for what is strangest, what is most unique or individual to the patient, because this will give the most accurate match to the remedy.

When the classical homoeopath grades the symptoms, five categories arise which range from the most individual to the most common. The top one is Strange, Rare and Peculiar; the next Mental and Emotional, because this level is the most individualistic, and forms the character of the human. The General level, which is the third category, refers to the organism functioning as a whole: 'I am cold', 'I am tired', rather than 'My hands are cold', which is the fourth category, the Particulars. The last category, the Common symptoms, is the lowest to the homoeopath but probably the most important to the doctor, as it enables him or her to group symptoms so disease labels can be applied, a process called diagnosis. To the homoeopath it does not help the selection of the remedy to know that the patient has aching limbs, or a runny nose in a cold. There are too many choices of remedy, so more information is needed to individualize the case and narrow down the choice. Homoeopathy cannot be other than individualistic.

ACTIVITY 7

Look over the questions you have written down.
Do you have any greater understanding of these?

ACTIVITY 8

Write down answers to the following questions and check your answers in the text.

1) What makes homoeopathy holistic?
2) How can we describe homoeopathy as a natural treatment?
3) Why do we say there is only one disease?
4) What function do symptoms perform?
5) Name five basic principles of homoeopathy.
6) What does 'Silica 30' mean?
7) In the history of disease, why are the most serious symptoms the last ones to occur?
8) What do the following words mean? The Glossary at the end of the course will help you.

    Remedy
    Prover
    Symptom picture
    Tincture
    Crude dose
    Succussion
    Symptom
    Allopathy
    Potency
    Dynamic

READINGS

Hahnemann S *The organon*, Paras 1–5
Kent J T *Lectures on homoeopathic philosophy*, Chs 1 & 2
Vithoulkas G *The science of homoeopathy*, Chs 1 & 2

ADDITIONAL READING (for interest only)

Campbell A *1984 The two faces of homoeopathy.* Jain, New Delhi
Coulter H *1973 The divided legacy.* North Atlantic Books, Berkeley, USA
Coulter H *1980 Homoeopathic science and modern medicine.* North Atlantic Books, Berkeley, USA
Illich I *1977 Medical nemesis.* Penguin, London
Ortega S *1980 Notes on the miasms.* The National Homoeopathic Pharmacy, New Delhi

LESSON TWO

The Vital Force

Headings: The Vital Force
The Homoeopathic Theory of Disease
The Maintaining Cause

Aims: This lesson is to introduce you to the basic principles of the vital force's action.

Objectives: To have some understanding of what is meant by 'the integrity of the whole';
To know the difference between the disturbance and the effects it produces (symptoms);
To recognize the role of predisposition, vitality and exciting cause in causing illness;
To identify some factors inimical to life;
To tell the difference between an exciting and a maintaining cause.

The Vital Force

Vitalism

It is not so much the Law of Similars, from which homoeopathy derives its name, as its attitude to vitalism that makes homoeopathy so distinctive. We can say to the patient that it is not the medicine, homoeopathic or otherwise, that cures, but the patient him or herself. The medicine only stimulates the body's own healing mechanism.

Paragraphs 9 and 11 of the *Organon* contain Hahnemann's thoughts on the matter. The organism is living matter that has direction and purpose. It grows, reproduces itself and repairs itself. These processes are automatic. The programme exists irrespective of human consciousness. Living matter has a fundamental mysterious energy that makes it very different from inorganic matter. The nature of this substance has eluded philosophers, but there is no difference in shape or chemistry between a living body and a dead body (before decay sets in), except that the living body has this mysterious energy. Hahnemann called it the *vital force* or *vital principle* and admitted that *we know nothing of it except its effects, the results of its actions.* Yet if this is the force that holds the organism together as a harmonious whole, then it is this force we must reach with our medicines; we would not be ill if all were well with the vital force, and if we cannot know the vital force itself since it is invisible and intangible, we must study its effects and know it by its actions – as we do with magnetism and electricity.

In order to apply medicines that affect its actions, we must ask how the vital force affects health. When all is well we see nothing. When the body is well, what do we feel? The absence of illness? Health? How do we recognize light if not by its absence? Health may be described as an absence of symptoms. *Certainly the presence of symptoms is a sign of ill health.* Hahnemann tells us (para 12) we can know nothing of illness but the symptoms produced. In health we see nothing of the vital force; in sickness we recognize its actions by studying the pattern and movement of symptoms caused by the reaction of the vital force.

We cannot see or feel the action of the vital force. We can look at the patterns of activity of the organism in health, and speak of some thing or plan that maintains integrity, but what is it that keeps the whole together? It is obviously more than the cohesive attraction of the molecules. There are well-trodden pathways of interaction that connect the parts of an organism, so there is a relationship between symptoms in disease. Once you see this there is a sense of a vibrant whole. It is an energy system. We speak of the strength of an energy field that keeps it together. But ... what is that strength? In music we can talk of the volume or intensity of a note, but this does not give the note its character or nature. We are back again into the realms of speculative

9

philosophy, or quantum physics! How do we measure human energy? What makes us what we are?

ACTIVITY 1 List five things you now know about the Vital Force.

Integrity of the Whole

The role of the vital force is to maintain the integrity of the whole. When the integrity of the whole is disturbed, the role of the vital force is to correct or recover that integrity. A spinning top knocked off balance may wobble, depending on how severely it is struck, but if its momentum is sufficient, it will continue to spin as if nothing had happened.

Here we have two of the three principles that determine the degree of ill health, namely vitality (momentum), and exciting cause (disturbance). The third factor in the equation is predisposition. It is the very nature or condition of the top that first allows it to spin. The method of expression of the life principle in an organism allows it to be. Dis-ease may be the sense that all is not well, that something is out of balance. The symptoms are the form that the disease takes (paragraph 14), but the real disease is the disturbance that challenges the integrity of the whole by affecting the vital force.

If we look at another model, we may understand a little more of the action of the vital force. If a stone is thrown into a still pond it creates a disturbance which spreads outwards from the point at which the stone entered. The ripples or waves move to accommodate the new demand on space, but in so doing they dissipate the energy created by the disturbance, so allowing the pond to return to normal as quickly as possible. This brings us to one of the most fundamental statements in homoeopathy: *symptoms are created to restore the patient to normal functioning* (para 12).

Symptoms Restore Normal Functioning

The vomiting or diarrhoea of food poisoning is an attempt by the body to expel the poison and so right itself. A high fever may be an attempt to make the body's environment unacceptable to bacteria. The heat and activity of the blood may also be seen as the intensified action of the vital force strengthening the energy field, or re-establishing its own nature. In the homoeopath's understanding it is the Vital Force that is disturbed in maintaining the integrity of the whole (para 11). As it gives, 'the reverbations that run through the organism are shock waves that spread the energy of the disturbance and so dissipate it'. This point of view becomes more dynamic when we consider that we are dealing with a living organism. How much are we just a result of reaction to our environment?

Disease: Resistance to Flow

Kent spoke of disease as being caused by resistance to the outward movement of the symptoms, i.e. to the correcting action to the vital force. If we stop the wave moving outwards it will gather force behind it to break through, or will sidestep into a less crowded space, temporarily in that local area increasing the energy of the disturbance so the patient feels worse. The longer the block exists, or the closer to the source of the disturbance, then the greater the energy of the disturbance and the more the patient feels un-ease. So we can say that *the intensity and severity of the symptoms* (the vital force's reaction) *depend on the severity of the disturbance and/or the vitality or ability of the vital force to react.*

Later we will see that this last is a very important statement, an understanding of which is necessary to help us in the accurate choice of potency.

ACTIVITY 2 Watch the action of water in a stream, how it speeds up (or increases force) as its channel is narrowed to get past obstacles.

What happens when you put an obstacle in the stream?

The Homoeopathic Theory of Disease

One Disease

Each Vital Force is Unique

If we have a concept of the vital force maintaining the integrity of the whole, and therefore health, it follows that disease can be no more than a disturbance or affliction of the vital force, which interferes with its activity to maintain harmony (para 1). It also follows that this is only one disease (para 12). How can there be more than one disease, if any disease is merely a disturbance of the harmony created by the vital force?

The real question is why symptoms have such varieties of patterns. The answer the homoeopath will give is that each one of us is unique. Each organism has different weaknesses and a different reaction to stress. Disturbance will manifest according to the lines of weakness in this organism, and all groups of symptoms will be related.

The homoeopath does not use disease labels as does the allopath, because *each vital force is unique in the patterns it produces*. When we are ill, we produce different patterns of illness. On the one hand, we each tend to succumb to certain types of illness, so we might be labelled a bronchitic, or prone to high fevers or digestive disturbances, etc. We are here talking of a constitutional type. Each has weak organs and succumbs when the vitality is lowered, or the assault on integrity is so severe as to affect the functioning of the vital force. Later we will see how the homoeopath uses this concept to improve the long-term health of a person. Now it is important to recognize that even in typhoid, or just a cold, there is an individualistic pattern to the symptoms.

In a cold epidemic in the office, 20 out of 30 people 'catch' it. Let us go into the office and see what is happening.

Why do 10 people not catch it if it is so virulent? We will come back to that question; let us keep it in mind. Twenty people have the cold, but they each have *their* cold, i.e. the usual pattern of symptoms familiar to each of them. Three have developed chest problems, but even here one is a dry chest which makes breathing painful; another has a tickly cough that bothers him especially when he lies down to sleep, then it restarts in the morning as he brings up yellow evil-smelling mucus; the last coughs up volumes of green phlegm continually, unless she goes out into the cool air. Whenever these three catch cold they commonly produce their own pattern, irrespective of which virus or bacteria, etc. Now the others are just as fascinating. They may just have runny noses, but the varieties are stupendous. One has thin discharge, whereas another's is thick; one has yellow, another green, and yet another has white; one has acrid discharge running out of the left nostril only, another has thick green only out of the right, and yet another has thick yellow in the morning that turns thin and white by afternoon, but also changes nostril continually. Ann in the corner has streaming eyes with her runny nose, whereas Jacqueline has a sore right ear; Maisie has a sore left nostril and an agonising pain when she gulps the empty air, but it's fine to gorge herself with her favourite chocolates as compensation. There's more . . . .

This is just a corner of the immensely rich homoeopathic garden, which henceforth will continue to astound with its variety, even if this little glance of details might start to put you off!

Predisposition

The homoeopath must ask where this variety comes from if the cold is the work of the same virus. This becomes a particularly significant question when Ann and Maisie etc. produce similar symptoms each time they have a cold, even when each epidemic has a different virus. The homoeopath's answer (and also that of Louis Pasteur) is to say that the virus/bacteria is not important, it is the soil that allows the germ to grow. When the vital force is afflicted it throws out a pattern of symptoms, each according to its own peculiarities. Even in an affliction such as typhoid or polio, where there is a distinct pattern of symptoms that enables the doctor to label this as a specific disease, the homoeopath will put aside the common disease symptoms in favour of the uniquely individual symptoms that enable us to reach this patient's vital force, and the remedy tailored precisely to its unique character.

The unique patterns of weakness are called *predispositions* by the homoeopath, i.e. *constitutional weaknesses that are predisposed towards certain patterns of disease*.

Two questions remain for us:

Why do some people not succumb to the epidemic?

What causes disease if not virus and bacteria?

The answer to both these questions is the same.

In a crowded room there is a great deal of noise, but we still hear the sound of our own name – it is our note. Vithoulkas explains it as *resonance*. The tuning fork responds to its own note; we do not hear German if we do not speak it – it disturbs us less if we're trying to concentrate. At a party or an evening class we will home in on those most like ourselves; we will see as excessive rudeness or bad taste those things with which secretly we ourselves most fear to be labelled. Relationships function on the principle of resonance. Some people never get colds because it is not their weakness. They may succumb rapidly to something else, but if a cold is not their weakness they will not answer to that note. If the *predisposition* does not exist, disease will not follow.

Vitality

Some diseases represent forces so inimical to life that almost all vital forces are affected, yet still some refuse to succumb. Diseases such as typhoid are an example of this, yet some still fail to be affected. Why? The predisposition is not sufficient: the vitality must also be lowered.

Many factors lower vitality. In the case of the epidemic it may be fear, or the burden of nursing the sick in the family, or of carrying on with the workload of absent colleagues. The patterns of symptoms we see in response to a flu epidemic may also appear without the epidemic, after stress or shock such as grief, i.e. spontaneously, irrespective of bacteria.

One comment needs to be made here concerning vitality: each day many of us already have present within our bodies the virus and bacteria that cause colds etc. but we do not succumb; however, lower our vitality and we do succumb, *if we have the predisposing weakness.*

Exciting Cause

Now, even when we have the weakness and a lowered vitality, most of the time we still do not become ill. The third ingredient is what the homoeopath calls *the exciting cause*: the vital force must meet that which disturbs its action, that which is inimical to life, that resonates to its own pattern of weakness. We may be fortunate that, despite feeling worn down, we do not meet our exciting cause, so we do not become ill but are restored by a good night's sleep, or a good meal or nice company. At other times we may not be so lucky.

ACTIVITY 3   Name three facts you now know about predisposition.
Give five examples of an exciting cause.

The Maintaining Cause

Even given a healthy vital force there are five things necessary each day for successful functioning. These are:

- Oxygen
- Water
- Food
- Sleep
- Exercise

The absence of any one of these factors will affect vitality in a detrimental manner. Usually we will recover quickly after small lapses, but if the organism is continually deprived significant lowering of vitality will weaken our resistance to exciting causes (disturbing factors) and make us more liable to become ill.

This type of disease requires treatment by drugs less than by a better, sounder daily regime. In other words, the patient's daily habits have created weaknesses which can best be remedied by better habits.

Sometimes, though, perhaps through no fault of our own, we are exposed daily to detrimental factors. For example, we may live in a damp basement. When we are healthy this is of no consequence, but after continual exposure we may begin to feel the effects because such an environment is basically unnatural and therefore unhealthy. If there is a predisposing weakness in the lungs it may be a very short time before ill health shows, and if we continue to live in the same environment it is possible we will become seriously ill. Medical treatment will be required and may prove useful, but no thorough cure can take place until we remove ourselves from the damp basement residence.

The damp basement in this example is a maintaining cause of disease, and when the maintaining cause is removed, cure automatically follows. Hahnemann calls this type of disease *pseudochronic* false disease, because it is not so much an attack on the vital force as a continual niggle, wearing down vitality. Much of the disease we see around us today is of this type because of environmental pollution (chemical, dirt, noise etc.), stressful lifestyles, poor diet, unclean air and water, 'high living' often accompanied by lack of sleep, and lack of exercise due to sedentary lifestyles.

ACTIVITY 4	Keep an account of your habits over 1 week. How many hours sleep do you get at night? What do you eat each day? What chemicals are artificially added ingredients in your food? How much exercise did you have each day? How much water do you drink each day? What are the impurities in the water? (The Local Water Board will give you a list of these.) If possible compare your pattern with that of an old person with rheumatism or arthritis, and also do a comparison with a young healthy child.

ACTIVITY 5	If you are using this course with a tutor you may find it useful to write a 1000 word essay on your understanding of the action of the vital force so far.

READINGS

Hahnemann S *The organon*, paras 6–19, 34–45, 272–274
Kent J T *Lectures on homoeopathic philosophy*, Chs 3, 4, 5, 8 & 9
Vithoulkas G *The science of homoeopathy*, Chs 3, 4 & 5

SELF-ASSESSMENT QUESTIONS	1)	Why do we study the fifth and sixth editions of the *Organon*?
	2)	Why are symptoms so important to a homoeopath?
	3)	Name the three factors needed before disease can occur.
	4)	Comment on your understanding of disease as a resistance to the flow of the vital force.
	5)	What is the one disease from which the organism can suffer?
	6)	Discuss in your own words what is meant by a predisposition. Give three examples.
	7)	Give two examples of a maintaining cause.

LESSON THREE

Resonance – The Law of Similars

Headings: Homoeopathy is the Law of Similars
The Dynamic Vital Force
The Law of Similars
The Similimum
The Total Symptom Picture
Amelioration and Aggravation
The Point of Change or Exciting Cause

Aims: This lesson will explain how the vital force becomes diseased, and therefore the mechanism by which it can be healed.

Objectives: To develop a concept of the organism as an energy unit;
To understand the role of a total symptom picture in representing the one disease;
To recognize an aggravation,
an amelioration, and
a point of change

Homoeopathy is the Law of Similars

It is from the Law of Similars that homoeopathy derives its name: like cures like. When the symptom picture produced by the patient is matched to a remedy that can produce the same symptom picture in a healthy person, cure is initiated. Vithoulkas has helped us to understand this in the language of modern science, in which it is called resonance.

The Dynamic Vital Force

Energy Affects Energy

Not all factors are capable of afflicting the vital force and disturbing the harmony it creates. The vital force responds only to factors which have some similarity or resonance to its own nature. This is a basic law of interaction in living organisms. Hahnemann recognized this process when he said that the vital force was of a 'dynamic nature', and could be affected only by some cause that was also of a 'dynamic nature' (para 16). He used the word 'dynamic' as we would use the word 'energy' today.

Thus, the vital force is primarily an energy. The cause of disease is seldom material; of course, if we fall off a ladder the material part of us may be affected, but local trauma is a special category of disease. When it happens to otherwise healthy people, it can be expected to heal in a short period of time without complications.

Orthodox medicine believes most infections to be caused by germs, whether bacteria, spirochaetes or viruses. A germ is a life form, an energy body, that can tune into the level of a human vital force. Special conditions must be required for this activity, since many of us carry a variety of harmful germs – in our mouth, anus, vagina, under our nails, on our skin – but seldom develop illness as a result. It begs the question as to the state of health of the more complex human life form, that it can be so affected by such a simple life form!

In taking this approach, homoeopathy does not sidestep the question left unanswered by the biologist, i.e. What is life? Ultimately, the biologist hesitates to reduce life to chemical reactions. When we talk of the human non-material form, we use words such as 'soul'. This is a gigantic leap in imagery which a good homoeopath should not be prepared to take. Hahnemann the scientist aimed not to speculate nor to theorize, but to stick to facts. So, if we accept the energy nature of the human organism, what does it mean?

15

Subtle Causes

We are so indoctrinated to believe that disease is caused materially that we ignore the many subtle causes that affect us. As homoeopaths we must learn to pay attention to these.

Psychotherapy teaches us about the complex integration that forms a human being. Most people develop strategy to survive which gives shape to personality. These adaptations then give rise to stresses and strains that predispose individuals to particular illnesses. Since these are usually of a mental and emotional nature, which is non-material, it would allow us to agree with Hahnemann that the only affliction of the vital force is dynamic in nature. Although true, this is an oversimplification.

Hahnemann labelled causes as 'morbific agents'. In modern language this means 'evil'. If you put aside moralistic hang-ups and ask what is meant by this, it is possible to translate it into the modern concept of 'negativity'. This can then apply to factors which are physical, mental, emotional, or even psychic. If we are negative of mind it may lead to a depression of the vitality, which is often followed by illness. The process is easily recognized when the emotion is great, as in grief, but it is a subtle process that surrounds us daily. Many modern psychological texts describe this, and promote the development of a positive attitude. Some useful thoughts on the subject appear in the introduction to Edward C. Whitmont's book *Psyche and Substance.*

Psychology also shows us that the individual is selective in what he or she reacts to in the environment. The individual is attracted to situations that resonate his or her specific needs or weaknesses, and is sustained or afflicted by such situations. A good Quaker term calls these situations that 'speak to our condition'.

ACTIVITY 1

You will need a bar magnet, some iron filings, a sheet of white paper, and a series of metal and other objects.
Magnetism is an energy; its source or field of action can be demonstrated by scattering iron filings on a white sheet of paper covering a bar magnet. A beautiful pattern is described.
What affects this energy field?
Experiment with different objects.
What common characteristics describe the objects that are affected by the energy field of the magnet?

The Law of Similars

It is necessary to be explicit as to how the vital force works.

If it is recognized that the vital force produces symptoms as a process of dissipating the energy of the disturbance, like the current in a stream, these symptoms will follow the line of least resistance, because that is the way energy moves! The symptoms produced by the vital force are those most likely therefore to restore health fastest. The vital force orders the symptoms in a way which will cause the least damage to the integrity of the whole. *Therefore in order to restore the patient to health in the most rapid gentle manner, we must use the medicine that can concentrate on exactly these symptoms.* The more exact the match between the symptoms the remedy can cause, and the symptoms now produced by the disturbed vital force, the greater the ability of the remedy to resonate with the sick person and affect their health. It is this application of the medicine that makes the medicine homoeopathic, not simply the fact that it is a potentized medicine.

Hahnemann (para 148) tells us that the effectiveness of the homoeopathic remedy is that it can create the same symptoms the vital force is already producing to quell the disturbance. Because of this the patient is cured faster, and usually more gently. He argues:

- That there can only be one disease;
- That the symptoms are a result of the vital force's action to quell the disturbance;
- That the homoeopathic remedy acts by increasing those same symptoms;
- That the medicine introduces an artificial disease that is stronger than the real disease;

- That the artificial disease is limited in time by the fact the medicine is limited in its action, being artificially induced;
- When the action of the medicine ends the disturbance comes to an end, and in time the symptoms recede and the vital force goes back to normal functioning.

This is a brilliant piece of logic which can be clearly demonstrated in the action of the medicine on the prover, and it can be seen repeatedly in homoeopathic cure. Also, this is the reason why homoeopathic medicines are absolutely safe: no homoeopathic medicine acts unless there is a resonance with the vital force of the patient, and a homoeopathic medicine acts on the vital force which, by its nature, has the ability to select the most relevant reaction pattern. Almost every homoeopathic prescription is curative because, if it resonates with the vital force then its action is to increase symptoms which the vital force has already produced in order to quell the disturbance.

A very important facet that makes homoeopathy very different from orthodox medicine is the control that can be exerted on the degree of action, by the use of potency. The homoeopathic remedy is merely a stimulant to the vital force – it does not cure the patient. The vital force cures the patient, and needs only to hear its note/sound to tune up further to do the job better. The homoeopath can control the quality of the note, its rate of vibration or energy, through the potency used. The homoeopath uses the minimum dose to achieve the change, then stands back to monitor whether the change is sufficient to cause cure. The Law of Cure then becomes a tool to assess the degree of change.

The Similimum

Homoeopathy seeks the similimum, which is *similar* in symptom picture to the pattern of the diseased patient (Fig. 3.1). That which is *exactly* the same is not homoeopathy but isopathy (see note to para 57 of the *Organon*) (Fig. 3.2).

In his footnotes, especially in the sixth edition, Hahnemann postulates that *the same*, isopathy, can only increase the disturbance. This of course makes sense. In terms of sounding the same musical note, the exact same note strengthens and prolongs the note already sounded. Although the similimum (Fig. 3.3) is close enough to the disturbance to enhance the symptoms, *the organism can only be affected by one disturbance*, and if there are two *it is the stronger that holds sway*.

The great strength of homoeopathy is that the potency or dose of the medicine can be selected to strengthen its impact on the vital force. It is essential that the medicine creates a stronger disease that is similar enough to resonate with the disturbed vital force to take over. Yet, because it is medically induced, the homoeopathically induced disturbance is limited in its duration. As its action ends, the patient is no longer disturbed because the disease symptoms are already destroyed, and the remedy symptoms disappear when its action finishes (Fig. 3.4).

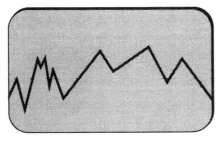

Fig. 3.1 A visual impression of the peaks and troughs of the patient's symptom picture.

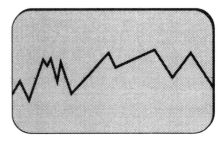

Fig. 3.2 The same – isopathy. A visual impression of the symptom picture of a remedy.

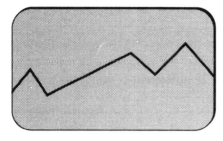

Fig. 3.3 The similimum.

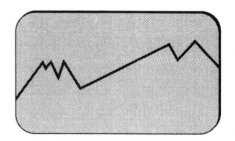

Fig. 3.4 A more exact similimum.

Figs 3.3 and 3.4 are similar. The remedy in Fig. 3.4 would be the most effective because it is the most similar, but that in Fig. 3.3 could also be expected to 'work'.

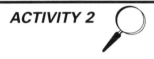

ACTIVITY 2

If you are familiar with the Materia Medica, briefly compare two or three remedies. Select areas of similarity, e.g. digestive symptoms of Nux Vomica, Colocynthis, Colchicum; Earaches of Pulsatilla, Belladonna and Chamomilla.
Show how they affect this area similarly, then pick out some symptoms that would distinguish each in these ailments.

Understanding the Opposite

If a spinning top is tilted it will reach the end of its orbit, but because it is moving (active) it rebounds back. In a pond, the ripple will spread out as far as it can, but it will rebound if it reaches the edge of the pond. The movement is contained within the limits of the pond just as the body has the limitations of its nature. If we increase the symptom eventually it will become its opposite.

The Chinese symbol for Yin and Yang (Fig. 3.5) very ably represents homoeopathic treatment. Each contains its opposite, and eventually, if we push reaction along the same line, in the same direction, we will get the opposite effect. The homoeopathic remedy increases the symptoms along the same line until the direction is exhausted and the organism recoils (Figs 3.6, 3.7). If we give a remedy with the opposite reaction, it could be argued that we create an equilibrium which could even be described as balance, but the object of therapeutics is not to cancel out the effect of symptoms but to create harmony by removing the disturbance and restoring calm. In Fig. 3.8 the equilibrium created is stressful, since it is a balance of forces pulling in different directions. Now there are two disturbances. Homoeopathy is based on fact and ruthless analysis of observation. In this section we are looking at the concepts behind the theory. Practical aspects need to be taught in a clinical setting, but it is worth noting that the first reaction

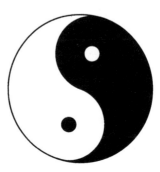

Fig. 3.5 Chinese symbol of Yin and Yang.

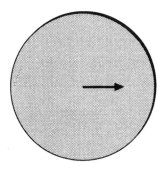

Fig. 3.6 The disturbance unbalances the organism, giving it a lean to one side.

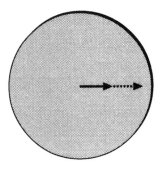

Fig. 3.7 By increasing the lean – i.e. the symptoms produced – it more speedily reaches the edge of its orbit and rebounds.

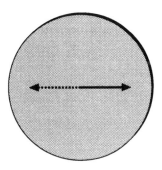

Fig. 3.8 If we push the top in another direction, we will introduce yet another factor of disturbance, even if the other direction is the opposite.

after homoeopathic treatment is that the patient feels better *even if the symptoms are worse*. The homoeopathic concept is that, after treatment, inner harmony is restored. Subjectively the patient should feel better because health – the integrity of the whole – is improved. To the homoeopath the removal of the symptoms is only part of the cure.

ACTIVITY 3 Find examples from your own experience to illustrate the homoeopathic process, e.g. the further east you go, the further west you are.

The Total Symptom Picture (TSP)

Just as there is only one disease and one disturbance of the vital force, (para 15), so there is only one pattern of symptoms. For closest resonance, the symptom picture of the remedy must match as closely as possible, in all aspects – breadth, length and height – the symptom picture of the patient. In other words, *all* the patient's symptoms must be taken into consideration in matching a remedy symptom picture. If the remedy affects the vital force it will affect every part of the organism. We say the *total symptom picture* must be considered (paras 17 and 18) (Figs 3.9 and 3.10). These diagrams are totally unscientific and are used to give a visual impression of the shape of the total symptom picture. Each peak may be used to represent a symptom, some being more important or intense than others and therefore reaching higher than others. In a 'real' patient there may be 20–40 symptoms. Figure 3.9 represents the TSP of the patient. Figure 3.10 gives the symptom picture of three remedies superimposed upon the TSP given in Fig. 3.9. Allegorically, we can see that Remedy B most closely traces the line of TSP. Remedy B is therefore the best-fit remedy or similimum.

When the homoeopath interviews and examines the patient to find the scope and detail of the symptoms, it is necessary to spend sufficient time to obtain the total

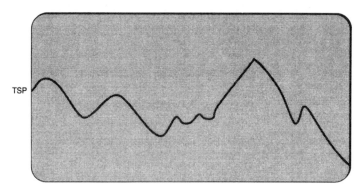

Fig. 3.9 Variations in the wave pattern produced by stimulus. Total symptom picture.

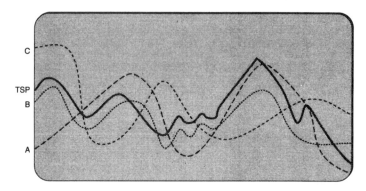

Fig. 3.10 Three remedy patterns superimposed on the TSP. Note that remedy A most closely traces the lines of the TSP, and is therefore the best-fit remedy.

symptom picture. Although it is possible to recognize the subject of the jigsaw when a few pieces are missing, it is very easy to make mistakes when only a few pieces are scrutinized. Just one important symptom may cause us to change our findings, to select another remedy. For example, the patient may have hit his thumb with a hammer, producing a red, hot swelling with a throbbing pain shooting up the arm. Our first inclination may be to reach for some Hypericum, but when we hear that the pain and swelling are better after cold applications it is likely we will give Belladonna instead.

Similarly we may have taken a case that involves severe head pains, suggesting a particular remedy. However, these symptoms may be produced by a patient who is very angry and cannot express the anger, or it may be that the symptoms arose after a vaccination or a head injury, or it may be they are the result of high blood pressure caused by malfunction of the kidneys. All of these symptoms might call for different remedies, even though the presenting symptoms of headache are the same. However, without eliciting the total symptom picture we may have misprescribed. Only with the total symptom picture can we decide on the best-fit remedy, because all symptoms are accounted for.

ACTIVITY 4   Once again, some exploration of Materia Medica will show examples of the above.

Amelioration and Aggravation

This is a convenient time to add some comments on these two concepts.

Aggravation

Because the homoeopathic remedy works by stimulating the vital force, it first increases the intensity of the symptoms. This is called the aggravation. There are some homoeopaths who would say the homoeopathic process of cure is incomplete without the aggravation, or even, 'How do you know cure has taken place if there is no aggravation?'. Others feel that the choice of potency can be accurately manipulated to lessen the aggravation; sometimes this is of great value. The best choice of potency would stimulate the vital force to cure without creating a surge of energy represented by sudden and greater intensity of the symptoms.

Amelioration

The amelioration, or the lessening of the intensity of symptoms, can be seen to follow the aggravation as the cure phase of the vital force's action is clearly entered.

The Point of Change or Exciting Cause

When a homoeopath looks at a case it may become obvious that there is a certain point at which ill health started. It was at this point that the vital force was disturbed or afflicted, and the symptom picture that developed after this was the attempt of the vital force to restore harmony. This point may have occurred minutes, hours or even years ago. Sometimes there may be more than one point of change, each with its corresponding symptom picture. For example, after moving from the south of France to the west of Scotland the patient developed a series of sore throats, which were treated with antibiotics. One winter after starting secondary school the patient developed pneumonia, and since then has had continual catarrh and a susceptibility to bronchitis. The homoeopath may treat the presenting picture of bronchitis reasonably well, but may not remove the susceptibility, until he or she goes back to the point of change, to ask what it was that disturbed the vital force – what it has not yet recovered from. Was it pneumonia, or what did happen when the patient went to a different school? Is it possible that the whole situation goes back much further, to when the patient moved to the west of Scotland, and was it the cultural change, or emotional shock, or a change in climate, or something else?

As well as the point of change, this event in the case history could be described as the exciting cause because it was here the vital force was disturbed. The cause to which it responded tells us a great deal about the vital force and its weaknesses, or those things with which it resonates. The homoeopathic remedy used must also be susceptible to this causation, and will create cure if it can resonate with the disturbance from which the vital force is trying to recover (see Figs 3.11 and 3.12).

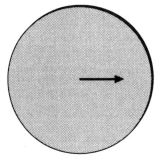

Fig. 3.11 The disturbed vital force moves out from its centre of gravity slightly.

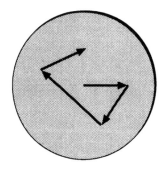

Fig. 3.12 How many times has the vital force been disturbed and so produced a slightly different symptom picture each time, one on top of the other chronologically? Where do the symptoms now present originate?

ACTIVITY 5 Note down some of your symptoms then put these in chronological order.
Attempt to identify any points of change or exciting causes.
If possible speak to others, and ask about symptoms they have.

READINGS

Hahnemann S *The organon*, paras 19–33, 53–57, 147–148
Kent J T *Lectures on homoeopathic philosophy*, Chs 10, 11, 12, 13 & 14
Vithoulkas G *The science of homoeopathy*, Chs 6 & 7

ADDITIONAL READING

Leonard G *1981 The silent pulse.* Wild Woodhouse, London
Dubos R *1965 Man adapting.* Yale University Press, New Haven

---

SELF-ASSESSMENT QUESTIONS

When you have answered these questions go back to the text to check your answers.
1) What are the differences between homoeopathy and isopathy?
2) Name three subtle causes that have affected your health.
3) Explain why the vital force must be regarded as an energy.
4) Give an example of local trauma and show why this does not disease the organism as a whole.
5) What do you understand by the term 'total symptom picture'?
6) The symptoms always aggravate after homoeopathic treatment. Discuss (in no more than 200 words).

LESSON FOUR

The Symptoms

'There is nothing morbid . . . that is curable which does not make itself known by means of marked signs and symptoms . . .'

The Organon, para 14

Headings: Definition of a Symptom
Types of Symptom
Hierarchy of Symptoms
How to Construct a Hierarchy
A Complete Symptom
Grades of Symptom in the Repertory

Aims: To understand the role of symptoms.

Objectives: By the end of this lesson you should be able to:
recognize the type of symptom;
recognize if a symptom is complete;
construct a hierarchy of symptoms;
recognize a grade of symptom in a repertory.

Definition of a Symptom

A symptom is a change in the body/mind which causes discomfort and shows an altered state of health in which the functioning of the body/mind becomes less efficient.

A symptom shows disharmony, or dis-ease, of the whole.

A symptom is produced by the vital force in the process of cure. Like the waves in a pond, the symptoms are used to dissipate the energy of the disturbance. Although the symptoms may appear higgledy-piggledy, there is a reason for each. Like running water, the vital force chooses channels of least resistance. First it will use the organs of excretion, but if these are blocked or insufficient it will find other routes. It will adapt other organs or systems such as the lungs or menstruation, then it will use weak organs.

There is system and pattern in the production of symptoms. To make sense of this system and pattern, let us first label some different types of symptom.

Types of Symptom

Symptoms can be classified in four different ways:

1. **Presenting**
   Prescribing
   Concomitant

   These label information given by the patient.

2. **Subjective**
   Objective

   This perspective becomes important because scientific procedure is usually seen as objective. Yet the patient's experience is also valuable, and this is subjective.

3. **Characteristic**

   In homoeopathic terms this describes the special pattern of a patient or remedy.

4. **Strange, Rare and Peculiar**
   Mental and Emotional
   General
   Particular
   Common

   These categories are used by the homoeopath to describe degrees of individuality and levels of activity of the vital force.

Presenting Symptoms *are those of which the patient complains, and so we are aware of these first.*

Mr Jones came into the clinic because he had a badly swollen elbow. This is his presenting symptom. Sometimes the homoeopath does not give much emphasis to the presenting symptom because it is only an external manifestation of the inner economy. However, it is important to Mr Jones, so the homoeopath must account for each presenting symptom and must find its position in the total symptom picture. A well-chosen remedy will deal with the presenting symptoms when it improves health and raises the vitality of the vital force.

Examples:
- You go to the dentist with toothache (presenting symptom), but it may be that the cause is an abscess.
- Pain in the ear (presenting symptom) may arise from inflammation of the mastoid area.
- Tightness in the chest area (presenting symptom) may focus the grief and distress a patient experiences after her mother dies.
- Duodenal ulcer (presenting symptom) may be caused by hurried eating to return to work, because the patient is insecure and anxious about his ability to complete the work satisfactorily.

Prescribing Symptoms *characterize the individuality and susceptibility of the patient.*

These are the most important symptoms because they enable us to identify the remedy. Remember, each remedy is unique in the way it affects patients, and we choose the remedy that matches the symptom picture produced by the patient. Kent describes prescribing symptoms as something that stops us in our tracks, making us hesitate because it is unusual, or out of the ordinary. It will not amaze us that a patient has a red face with a high fever, but our curiosity is stimulated if she has a red face only when she tries to lie down. Such a symptom is valuable to the homoeopath because it is individual. Few remedies have this unusual variation, so it is easier to single out a remedy. All prescribing symptoms are out of the ordinary and unexpected.

Examples:
- Sweating occurs only on the head, or only on uncovered parts.
- The cold feet are blue and sweaty.
- The pain of the piles continues for at least 2 hours after the stool is passed.
- Despite the heat of the fever the patient refuses to drink.
- Sweat is absent in the child's high temperature.

Concomitant Symptoms *accompany and are associated with other symptoms.*

Sweating is commonly associated with fever, but when it occurs with diarrhoea or pain it is a concomitant symptom. In a remedy such as Antimonium Crudem, gastric problems are associated with skin eruptions.

Examples:
- Headache accompanied by nausea.
- Swelling accompanied by stinging pains.
- Copious urination accompanied by cold feet.
- Numbness of the fingers and toes, accompanied by copious urination.

ACTIVITY 1   Give at least five examples of prescribing, presenting and concomitant symptoms.
Go back and check your examples with those in the text.

Objective Symptoms *are observable by someone other than the patient.*

The whole range of tests, diagnostic procedures and instrumentation in modern medicine have been created to discover objective symptoms. The doctor uses these symptoms to build up a pattern to which disease labels are applied – these then become common symptoms, of course. In the absence of objective signs, the doctor is unwilling to apply a label, and so cannot easily tell the patient what is wrong.

Subjective Symptoms *are felt only by the patient.*

Subjective symptoms are therefore not verifiable scientifically. If you feel hot, tired or thirsty, who can tell if you are right? Can I tell you how thirsty you are? Or how cold you are? Or how hungry you are? There are no instruments to measure these factors.

Of course, we are reliant on the patient telling the truth about subjective symptoms, and we are reliant on his or her ability to describe such symptoms accurately; this is another matter we will deal with under case-taking procedures.

One valuable aspect of the subjective symptom to preventive medicine lies in the ability of the patient to *feel* ill long before overt pathology develops. On the subjective level the patient's vital force may be less disturbed, and thus more easily cured.

The homoeopath is equally at home with both sets of symptoms, and indeed usually puts greater emphasis on the subjective symptoms because many of these represent the mind of the patient, which is the most evolved and individual part. These symptoms are not unscientific to the homoeopath, because they are present in the provings of the remedies, so it is a simple matter to include them in the symptom picture without worrying about their lack of objectivity. Some of the provings were done almost 200 years ago, and you can read the documentation or do a proving of your own and still come up with the same symptoms!

ACTIVITY 2 From your own experience, give five examples each of objective and subjective symptoms.

Characteristic Symptoms *may apply to the patient or the remedy; usually we think of them as forming a remedy's distinctive symptom picture.*

When ill, each patient produces symptoms which are repetitions of previous illnesses, so illness is not self-contained and omnipotent but is manifest by the individual according to his or her own pattern of weakness (predisposition). For example, Mrs Auld may have nausea and/or dizziness precede any illness, whether it be a cold, food poisoning, typhoid, etc., and this characteristic weakness may make her prone to motion sickness and may be prevalent when she has less sleep than normal. Another example may involve 20 patients who all need the remedy Nux vomica, even though they have different illnesses: one may be arthritic, another have croup, another heartburn, one have high blood pressure, yet all are characterized as impulsive, easily angered people who all suffer from pressing pain on the vertex of the head after eating rich foods. The last group of symptoms is characteristic of the remedy Nux vomica, and there is no physiology connecting them in the illnesses mentioned. Occuring as a pattern they form the Materia Medica, the symptom picture characteristic of a remedy.

ACTIVITY 3 Give at least ten examples of characteristic symptoms from the remedies you have studied.
Nash's Materia Medica deals almost entirely with characteristic symptoms, whereas von Lippe and Allen put them in heavy black type.
Do not forget to name the remedy.

The fourth classification will be dealt with under the hierarchy of symptoms.

Hierarchy of Symptoms

The hierarchy of symptoms is most fully developed by Kent. The basic premise is that some symptoms are more important than others. Some symptoms are more expressive of individuality and uniqueness, and therefore enable a more precise match to the symptom picture of a remedy. Some symptoms indicate a deeper disturbance of the vital force.

The Hierarchy

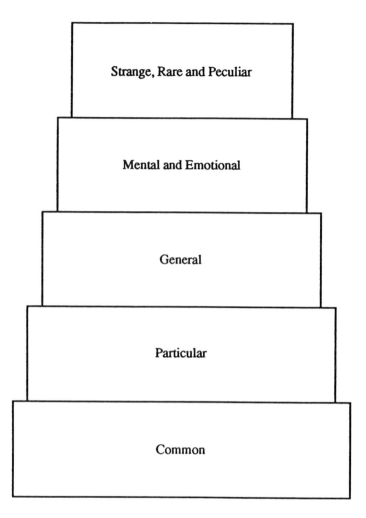

Strange, Rare and Peculiar (S, R & P)

These are just what the name suggests. They are *rare* and *uncommon*. During the provings few provers produced S, R & P symptoms: these are only produced when the remedy being proved is strongly resonant to the prover's vital force. Thus when S, R & P symptoms are present they point to so few remedies that, when matched with the patient's total symptom picture, one of these remedies will have a profound effect. An S, R & P symptom is therefore of great value.

S, R & P symptoms may come from any of the other groups except that containing the Common symptoms. Examples on the mental and emotional level may be:

- Laughs at serious things;
- Dreams that are prophetic;
- Hysteria better after eating;
- Thinks there is a man in bed with her (when there is not);
- Worse from consolation after suffering grief.

On the general level, examples might be:

- Sleepy in the daytime, sleepless at night;
- Faints after a bowel movement;
- Sweats only on the left side;
- Much worse for first movement but better for continued motion.

There are many S, R & P symptoms at the particular level. In the head we might have:

- Feels head is made of wood;
- Teeth feel too long.

Elsewhere examples might be:

- Purple halo around the urine;
- Sensation of a ball rising from the stomach to the throat.

H. A. Roberts has collected S, R & P symptoms in a book called *Sensations as if. . . .*
See Bibliography.

The beginner often confuses S, R & P symptoms with intensity of sensation. If someone is so afraid of dogs that he or she screeches and rushes hysterically from the room when a dog enters, the fear is intense! If a patient is afraid of needles, it may be he or she has had a very nasty experience in the past to which the fear is linked. If there is no past and no reason, we must consider this fear as an S, R & P symptom, especially when the patient faints at the sight of any sharp implement. There are reasons to be afraid of dogs – they can be dangerous animals, they have a mind of their own. Needles are inanimate objects over which we have control.

Mental and Emotional

These refer to all emotions, to temperaments, to disturbances of the will and understanding. Dreams are included, as are delusions, sleep-walking or talking, fears, preference for company or solitude, embarrassment, forgetfulness, laziness.

ACTIVITY 4

The first section of Kent's Repertory is called the Mind, and a glance through this will give you a good idea of the variety of mental and emotional symptoms. It is written in American English of the last century, so you may have to examine the meaning of the language very carefully.

The mental and emotional symptom is put so high in the hierarchy because it represents the character of the individual, i.e. it labels that which makes us stand out most clearly as humans and as individuals. It is the most highly evolved part of human society, distinguishing us from animals, plants and minerals. It represents the most complex part of our organism and, therefore, if deranged shows the deepest disturbance of the vital force, since such a derangement strikes deeply at our very nature.

All M/E symptoms are subjective but not all subjective symptoms are M/E. Some subjective symptoms are on the level of sensation, and it is these that appear first in any disorder, i.e. the feelings of dis-ease.

Some M/E symptoms are part of the temperament of character, and will help form a picture of the constitutional remedy. Others, such as irritability, may be a passing and understandable response to disease.

M/E symptoms put us into the realms of moral judgements of character and personal preferences and/or culture patterns. It is important that the homoeopath knows him or herself very well, in order to eliminate personal preferences. An ability is also needed to see the patient within his or her own culture. We are looking for individuality, and so must take out the norm. What choices are available to the patient? What factors give rise to such behavioural patterns? Under what conditions is the symptom produced? The homoeopath is not a psychologist, but must have an understanding of people!

General Symptoms

These refer to the body as a whole, and to metabolic processes such as digestion, excretion, sweating, sleeping, menstruation. In Kent's Repertory some of these have their own sections, e.g. Sleep, Perspiration. Others, such as menstruation, urination and appetite, are found under the relevant parts. Most general symptoms are found in the section called Generalities.

A general symptom is indicated when a patient speaks of 'I . . .' (I am tired, I am cold, I am feeling faint, I am nauseous) rather than the parts (my stomach is nauseous??? my arm is tired of writing, my feet are cold). When three or more parts share the same modality, that modality is elevated to the level of a general symptom. For example, left-sidedness becomes a general symptom if the warts are on the left side, the rheumatism is in the left knee, the headache is over the left eye.

GENERAL SYMPTOMS INCLUDE MOST EXCITING AND MAINTAINING CAUSES, WHICH ARE THE TRIGGER FACTORS THAT DISTURB THE VITAL FORCE AND WEAKEN IT SO THAT ILLNESS MAY FOLLOW. COLDS, SORE EARS AND SORE THROATS ARE OFTEN CAUSED BY EXPOSURE TO COLD WEATHER, SO THE GENERAL SYMPTOM IS WORSE IN COLD WEATHER.

Particular Symptoms

These refer to separate parts of body, such as the hands, feet, heart, eyes.

If the symptom of a part is well defined, with qualities of time, location, sensation and modality, it gains in importance within the hierarchy or, if it is S, R & P, it may even go right to the top of the list. Usually, however, the particular symptoms are of less importance because they do not reflect the whole of the organism, and by their physiological nature they are restricted in the degree to which they can represent individuality. There are only a limited number of ways in which the structure and function of an organ can break down.

Some particular symptoms are more important than others because they may show greater disturbance of the organization of the whole organism. When the vital force throws any disturbance as far from the centre as possible, this may result in a wart on the finger, which is relatively unimportant although an indication of disorder. 'Palpitations every time food is consumed' are an unnatural accompaniment to an act necessary for survival. A vital organ is acting out of turn, showing greater disturbance in the harmony of the whole. It is a much more important symptom than a wart, and is in fact strange, rare and peculiar. We will study this more thoroughly in the lesson on the Law of Cure.

Many presenting symptoms are particular symptoms, because we are not taught in our culture to see the body as a whole but as physical and divided into separate units. An allopathic approach to medicine based on biochemistry can often detect nothing wrong if there are no physical symptoms in the parts; conversely, biochemical abnormalities may be present in the absence of physical symptoms.

Examples:
- A callus on the left index finger;
- Excess sugar in the urine;
- Dry brittle hair that splits easily;
- Vomit of glairy grey mucus;
- Varicose veins since last pregnancy.

Common Symptoms

These are associated with disease patterns and are used by the allopath to diagnose 'diseases' such as the common cold, diabetes, acne, duodenal ulcer, measles and schizophrenia.

High sugar content in the blood is a diagnostic sign of diabetes; if this is found in tests it will limit the disease labels that the doctor can apply to the patient's illness. In the homoeopathic hierarchy of symptoms these common symptoms go to the bottom of the list, because they have no individuality: they arise from the pathophysiology of the tissue or organ involved. There is a limit to the number of ways the tissue can break down. The homoeopath will use these patterns, and needs to know them because we also treat the physical body! A knowledge of the patterns enables us to do two things: to know that which is not common, i.e. individual, and to predict the progress of the disease so we know the degree of disturbance of the vital force, and can therefore better select a potency and monitor the progress of the remedy in restoring order.

If you have a runny nose with a cold there is nothing for the homoeopath to prescribe on. If there is green mucus coming out of your left nostril only in the morning, there are three bits of individuality: greenness, left-sidedness and worse in the morning. Now the homoeopath has a case, and information to match to the symptom picture of a remedy.

Examples:
- Pain down the left arm in a heart attack;
- Burning pain in the epigastric area with a gastric ulcer;
- Opisthotonos with an increase of cerebrospinal fluid, as in meningitis;

- Sudden fatigue and weakness in a diabetic;
- Inflammation improved by cold compresses.

ACTIVITY 5 Look at the following list. Sort out these symptoms into five categories, and then place them into the table below.

Sensation of blood boiling in the arteries	All symptoms better after eating
Mental symptoms better after eating	Talks to himself
Chilly, lack of vital heat	Weepy before menses
Jealous	Cold clammy skin with internal burning
Sings in her sleep	Cannot bear to be looked at
Hissing noises in ear	Limbs ache in flu
Limbs ache	Apathy
Swollen cervical glands, left side	Sweats every other night
Painless swelling in the tonsils	Sneezing in hay fever
Laughter alternating with tears	Ulceration of the right leg
Bashful	Selfish
Frank and outspoken	Redness of lips, nose and eye margins
Mother indifferent to the welfare of her children	Shrieks before convulsion
Speaks quickly and incoherently	Sensation of a ball rising from the abdomen to the throat
Desires salty food	Throat pain extending to ear
Walks in sleep	Worse before menses
Metallic taste in mouth	Constipation
Worse before a thunderstorm	
Headache worse in a stuffy room	

S, R & P	Mental and Emotional	General	Particular	Common

Check these with the examples given earlier

How to Construct a Hierarchy

Case –
♀
8 yrs

Introverted since involved in an accident 16 months ago which she felt she caused. Fatigued easily. Chilly. Sits sucking her thumb. Flies into a rage when the accident is mentioned. Blond hair. Hides behind her mother on entering a room where a stranger is present.

The symptoms above have been collected from a patient and form the 'case'. The first step in making sense of them is to label each according to type of symptom. When we have done this a pattern of importance will start to emerge. We help formulate this by then arranging the symptoms into relevant hierarchical groups.

STEP ONE – **Labelling the type of symptom**

Symptom	*Type*	*Reason*
Introverted since involved in an accident 16 months ago which she felt she caused	M/E	The active word is introverted, describing a mental state

Symptom	Type	Reason
Easily fatigued	General	It is the whole body that is fatigued
Chilly	General	The heating mechanism is a metabolic process
Sits sucking her thumb	M/E	*What* sucks the thumb??? NO! *Who* sucks the thumb? Answer: the person
Flies into a rage when the accident is mentioned.	M/E	Once again it is the person who flies into a rage
Blond hair	Particular	This is a physical characteristic
Hides behind her mother on entering a room where a stranger is present	M/E	This is something the person does

In the example in this lesson I have made things slightly easier for you by grouping each symptom into a sentence. However, the first sentence actually contains two symptoms: the second, guilt, is only implied. I have done this deliberately because in a homoeopathic case you cannot make assumptions. You must have evidence for taking a thing implied as the real thing. To do so could cause you to prescribe on the wrong symptom picture. Thus part of the professional training is to evaluate the quality of the data given by the patient. Ask, what do you really know?

At present take each symptom as it is given. You will find, especially if you are working in a group, that there are plenty of different perspectives from which to view the data. The homoeopath has to learn to see all possible interpretations during the case-taking, and learn to ask questions that will clarify each symptom. I cannot overemphasize this.

At present take each symptom as it is given. Do not speculate.

STEP TWO – **put each symptom into a group**

S, R & P		
M/E	Introverted since involved in an accident 16 months ago which she thought she caused Sits sucking her thumb Flies into a rage when the accident is mentioned Hides behind her mother when entering a room where a stranger is present	
General	Easily fatigued	
Particular	Blond hair	
Common		

STEP THREE – **select which is the most important symptom within each group**

In the clinic it is unusual to find a perfect hierarchy which has one symptom above the other: often two or three symptoms may share importance. So, what we are doing here is a little artificial, but it is a very useful exercise to clarify your thinking.

Another difficulty, which has already been mentioned, will soon arise: our experience causes us to interpret symptoms in different ways. In a clinical situation, the total symptom picture and the context of each symptom favour one interpretation rather than another. Ambiguity arises in studying paper cases, especially such short ones as these. In other words, you may come up with different answers from mine because your experience weighs the evidence differently. Almost all the cases used here come from a clinical setting, so there is a definite loading that I am trying to represent.

M/E	1)	Flies into a rage when the accident is mentioned
	2)	Introverted since the accident, which she thinks she caused
	3)	Hides behind her mother when entering a room where a stranger is present
	4)	Sits sucking her thumb
Generals	5)	Chilly
	6)	Easily fatigued
Particular	7)	Blond hair

Why was this Order Adopted?

There appears to be an exciting cause – the accident – since when the symptom picture has changed and the child is introverted and flies into a rage. I have put 'flies into a rage' first because it is the most active of the two: introversion is the ongoing mental state from which she erupts into rage.

Hiding behind Mum is not connected to the accident and is common behaviour in a younger child, but this one is 8 years old so it is a prescribing symptom.

Thumb-sucking shows more immature behaviour but is not as restrictive as hiding behind Mum, so it comes last of the M/E symptoms.

Both the general symptoms indicate a lowered vitality. Fatigue is the more expected of these, and chilliness appears with lowered vitality only in certain patients, so it is put first as being more individual.

Blond hair is the least useful symptom to indicate individuality.

There are ten cases at the end of this lesson for you to work on yourself.

A Complete Symptom

When the patient tells of a symptom usually only a fraction of the information is conveyed. Mr Jones may complain of a sore elbow, but this is a particular symptom and its does not have enough individuality to be of value as a prescribing symptom, although there may be more information that would increase its value. Through further questioning each symptom can be explored further to *complete the symptom*. Questioning may find out more about the following:

- Time
- Location
- Sensation
- Modality
- Intensity

Time

The time when the symptom first arose may tell us more about the weak spots or predispositions of the vital force, and may be most valuable as an indicator of that to which it is resonant. For example, Mr Jones may get his sore elbow after he has cleaned the windows or the car. In itself this tells us little except that the elbow is weak and worse for exertion (vigorous use). However, it would be of greater value if we could say that the elbow has been sore on exertion since it was injured, or because it is his right elbow and overused since he broke his left arm (he is left-handed). Now we have more of a three-dimensional picture. Also, it may be that the discomfort began after a soaking – maybe he fell in the river, or was caught in very heavy rain and chilled – or after an argument with his boss or his girlfriend. The time is the point at which the symptom started or was caused. Often this is the *exciting cause*, the trigger to which this particular vital force reacts or is resonant. It may be that there is a *maintaining cause*, an ongoing exposure to detrimental environmental factors. Usually there is a build-up, so the maintaining cause is less obviously related to TIME.

The case is treated differently if there is a maintaining cause. A maintaining cause continually wears down vitality but, once removed, the body recovers, so the removal is a major part of the treatment. The exciting cause is a weakness in the vital force, so removal is only possible when the weakness is corrected through medication.

Location

The location of each symptom gives an idea of the accuracy and precision necessary in homoeopathic prescribing. If the patient has a headache, where is the pain? Above the right eye, or the left? Above the eye reaching backwards to the occiput, or extending from one eye to the other, from left to right or from right to left? Occipital region, or just starting there and extending over the left side, or the right? From the temple extending to the jaw? The exact location can lead to a quicker selection of the remedy, or to a closer fit with the symptom picture.

Sensation

The sensation of a symptom is subjective. It may cover such strange, rare and peculiar symptoms as that of a worm crawling up the throat, of blood boiling in the veins, or a pain that feels like red-hot needles. The psychologist may put this down to the vivid imagination of the patient. However, these symptoms can be found in the homoeopathic Materia Medica, the lists of remedy symptoms recorded in provings as long ago as 200 years. On taking a homoeopathic remedy in a proving dose many people will produce these same symptoms exactly. So, the homoeopath notes the sensations experienced by the patient and uses them to find a best-fit remedy, or Similimum.

The most common sensation experienced with a symptom is pain. This is entirely subjective, yet it cannot be dismissed as it is part of the body's alarm system. There are many studies of pain, mostly looking at its intensity and source with a view to better control. The many varieties of the actual sensation give the homoeopath a rich source for individualizing the symptom. Pain can be burning, stabbing, throbbing, pressure, inwards or outwards, bursting, like a constricting band, a heavy dull ache or a shooting pain, or it may sting. In Kent's repertory there are over 100 pages listing different types of head pain.

Modality

The modality of a symptom is what makes it better (>) or what makes it worse (<). Sadly, many people today simply banish pain with an aspirin, without looking to see what is indicated by the pain or without trying some of the simple old remedies, such as hot or cold compresses. Sometimes the best remedy is to remove themselves from a stuffy atmosphere, or to refrain from coffee, chocolate or whatever. What makes the symptom better or worse can help differentiate a remedy, or may give rise to S, R & P symptoms.

When more than one symptom has the same modality, that modality becomes a general symptom. It may still remain a modality, but we must ask if this is not a cause rather than merely a 'worse from', i.e. is it a weakness of the vital force, a trigger factor or exciting cause? If the modality is really causative it goes under the Time section. This distinction is important later when you start to use the Repertory to find remedies linked to specific symptoms, because you will find the entry in different sections.

Now, let us look again at Mr Jones' elbow:
It may be that the elbow has been sore since he injured it (*TIME*)

- and the pain is inside the right elbow (*LOCATION*)
- and may be described as shooting (*SENSATION*) towards the wrist (*LOCATION*)
- but it is better for hot applications (*MODALITY*)
- and for rest (*MODALITY*).
- However, it is prone to be worse when the weather is damp and cold (*MODALITY*).

Now we should be able to find a remedy more suited to Mr Jones' individuality. However; the elbow is only part of Mr Jones; he may be irritable with pain, and this response leads to a fuller picture containing M/E symptoms.

Intensity

Often there is a group of symptoms – sore throat, sore head, distended abdomen, swollen cervical glands and weepiness. There may be six, 12, or even 20 remedies that fit all these symptoms, but it may be that only one of these has cervical glands most pronounced. Another three remedies may have the headache most pronounced, and yet another may have the abdominal distension most pronounced. Such pronouncement, or *intensity*, forms a characteristic pattern, and knowing the emphasis given to symptoms within a remedy picture enables us to select the remedy more accurately.

The *intensity* of a symptom, especially when it is pain, may cause us to give that symptom prior consideration in another way. Some particular symptoms may indicate a medical emergency, such as appendicitis or meningitis, and these should be dealt with promptly to maintain life!

ACTIVITY 6   The Generalities section of Kent's Repertory contains many exciting causes.
List at least ten of these.

ACTIVITY 7   Write down, in as much detail as possible, the description of a headache you have experienced.
Ask at least three other people to describe their headache in the same detail.
You should find a considerable amount of variety.

ACTIVITY 8   For each of the following symptoms, give examples of:

time
location
sensation
modalities

and give some indication of intensity.

Ulcer on the leg	Breathlessness
Constipation	Back pain
Menstrual pain	Cold feet
Skin rash	Insomnia
Sore throat	Ravenous hunger
Blurred vision	Fainting
Migraine	High temperature
Cough	Sadness (depression)

Grades of Symptom in the Repertory

In most repertories there are three grades of symptom, represented by three different typefaces. These grades are devised from the provings of the remedies.

When a remedy is written in **bold black type** it means that the symptom was present in almost all the provers after they had taken the remedy. This same symptom is therefore highly marked and most characteristic in the symptom picture of a patient who needs that remedy.

Italic type is used when a large group of provers produced that symptom and it is known from clinical experience that the remedy has cured that symptom.

Ordinary type refers to a low occurrence of that symptom when the remedy was proved. Further provings or clinical experience may upgrade the symptom, otherwise it may not be significant at all in the symptom picture of the remedy.

ACTIVITY 9 Organize the following groups of symptoms into a hierarchy.

1) Flushes of heat upwards. Pains in joints move about at night. Red face with distended veins. Hot dry throat < eating sweet things.
Tickling cough. Thick rust-coloured sputum.
Empty sensation in the abdomen. Feels paralysed and unable to move.
Cannot bear anyone walking about in the room.

2) Backache worse after lifting things, better with rubbing and heat.
Constipation, with hard dry stools. Sweats on face while eating. Worse fasting. Worse after cold food and drink. Worse before menses. Thirst for large quantities. Weeps without cause.

3) Epistasis when menses absent. Black blood forms long threads (from nose). Nausea in the evening. Numbness on the right side. Dissatisfied with job. Anger before lunch. Anxiety prevents sleep.

4) Sudden unaccountable fear. Restlessness (mental). Worse while alone. Desire alcohol, especially brandy. Wakes 4 a.m. with anxiety. Limbs cold. Urine scanty and burning. Colic. Abdominal pain, burning > hot applications (e.g. hot-water bottle). Simultaneous vomiting and diarrhoea. Loathing of food.
Nausea even with the smell of food.

5) Convulsions, shrieks beforehand. Stiffness of neck with convulsions < hot baths. High temperatures. Dry heat and sweating alternate. Drowsy. Thirstlessness > cold applications. Irritable when roused.

6) Dry teasing persistent cough. < Breathing in < in a warm room < lying down.
Desires open air. Tearful. Warts on fingers of left hand. Fear of dogs. Fear of men.

7) Apathetic and indifferent. Tongue feels cold. Cold exterior with internal burning. Bluish pallor around the mouth. Swollen parotid glands. Gums bleed. Teeth feel loose. Putrid flatulence. Itching and burning of private parts. Great desire for fresh air. Hands puffy.

8) Peevish, whiny, dislikes work. Running sores behind the ears. Foul odour of breath. Burning pains in the abdomen. Excoriation of flexures and sweaty parts. Headache, with pressing pains on the vertex. Head feels numb and empty. Music saddens and causes to weep. Obesity.

9) Weak memory. Capricious appetite, rejects at the sight and smell of food. Hydrothorax. Stiff neck. Bowel movements painful. Stools jellylike with blood and mucus. Colic > bending double. Urine hot. Joints painful, red and hot. Very sensitive. Flies into rage on exposure to strong light.

READINGS

Review Hahnemann S *The organon*, paras 6–8, 14–17, 27, 153
Read Kent J T *Lectures on homoeopathic philosophy*, Chs 6, 10, 32, 33
Review Vithoulkas G *The science of homoeopathy*, pp. 190–195

LESSON FIVE

The Action of the Medicine

Headings: What is a Medicine?
Finding the Field of Action of a Medicine
The Action of a Medicine on the Vital Force
The Self-Limiting Action of the Medicine
Susceptibility
The Speed of Action of a Medicine
Summary

Aims: In this lesson we will look again at the vital force, but this time we will consider how its activities are affected by a medicine. It will contain revisions of Lessons 2 and 3.

Objectives: By the end of this lesson you should be able to:
determine the conditions under which a medicine will act in a state of disease;
understand the concept of susceptibility to the action of a medicine;
understand the effect of repeat doses of the medicine.

What is a Medicine?

If disease is no more than an alteration in the state of health, and cure is no more than a rectification of this, then *a medicine is a substance that can alter the state of health*. It can act with the vital force to create health or disease. In the *Medicines Act* (UK Act of Parliament) a medicine is defined as a substance given with the intention of cure.

Orthodox medicine does not accept that a medicine has two actions, but this is one of the fundamental tenets of homoeopathy regarding the nature of a medicine. How could the homoeopath justify giving a medicine that increases the patient's symptoms if it were not clear that the resolving of the situation was the next action of that same medicine?

Exactly how does a medicine affect the health of an organism? How do we determine which symptoms a medicine will affect?

ACTIVITY 1   The words drug, remedy and medicine are used interchangeably.
Can you find a difference between these three?

Finding the Field of Action of a Medicine

In paragraph 18 of the *Organon* Hahnemann tells us that each medicine is different in its properties, as each plant and mineral is different. To discover the character of each individual medicine (para 119), it is necessary to give the medicine to healthy individuals until symptoms are developed, i.e. until it affects the health of those individuals. This process is called a *proving*, and it produces in the prover those symptoms to which the medicine has resonance, i.e. which it can cause and can cure.

Through the provings, Hahnemann discovered that every medicine has two actions. He noted that Cinquona (from which quinine is derived) aided the patient suffering from malaria, and could not dispute this, so he wanted to find out *how* it worked. He took the medicine himself to observe the action closer at hand. When he, who did not have malaria, developed symptoms similar to that disease, he realized that a medicine which could cure a sick person could cause the same symptoms in a healthy person.

Hence he could give a medicine to healthy individuals to find out what symptoms it produced and by turning this around he could then give that medicine to sick people with the symptoms that medicine could cause.

To increase the accuracy of the proving, it is crucial to give the medicine to very healthy persons who are free of disturbances (symptoms) – the ripple pattern is best seen in the still, undisturbed pond! It follows that it is also necessary to restrict diet, habit, environment, strong emotions and other factors influencing the internal environment, if all variables are to be eliminated and the action of the medicine seen clearly. Of course there is a limit as to how far such non-contamination is possible. How can the constitutional predispositions of the prover be eliminated? These will affect his or her reactions to the medicine, but no two patients are alike, and considering that the remedy will only act on that which it has resonance, any of the changes in the prover's health will still reflect those changes the medicine is capable of making on the organism. Lesson 10 will deal with provings in more detail.

The great virtue of homoeopathic provings is that the potentized remedy produces a great range of symptoms, including Mental and Emotional as well as General and Particular types of symptom. It reaches every level of the organism. How can this be?

ACTIVITY 2

The nature of something is how it can be expected to behave.
Describe the nature of a piece of granite, a rose, a commuter waiting on a late train.
Define in your own words what is meant by nature.
How did you find out the nature of the granite, the rose and the commuter?

The Action of the Medicine on the Vital Force

The initial disturbance of the vital force is invisible. Disease itself is invisible and only makes itself known to us, like electricity and magnetism, by its effects. It is only when the symptoms appear that the disease becomes visible. Similarly, the action of the homoeopathic medicine on the vital force is only visible by its effects – by the symptoms produced in the proving, for example. Allopathic research into the action of drugs explores the chemical reactions created by those drugs in certain parts of the body. Allopathic diagnosis of disease determines which chemical actions in the body have been altered, and therefore which drugs are needed to change the reaction. The homoeopathic reaction is more than chemical.

As stated already, Hahnemann showed that the homoeopathic medicine is effective because it acts like the disease to disturb the vital force; he said it produced an artificial disease. In the proving the prover is healthy, so the action of the medicine is clearly to disturb the vital force producing 'dis-ease'. The symptoms are produced to quell this dis-ease, or spread the energy of disturbance. In a sick person the remedy does exactly the same. It further disturbs the vital force, increasing the symptoms produced, but since these symptoms are produced to spread the energy of the disturbance this action speeds up the second action of the medicine, which is to cure the disease or disturbance in the patient.

The body can only have one disease, one pattern of disturbance, no matter how many facets there are to this. There is only one vital force, one organism, and it works as a whole, not divisively. Throw stones into the pond: how many ripple patterns are there?

If a stronger disease is introduced it will supplant the old disease: a pebble thrown into the pond will create gentle ripples, but huge waves will obliterate the gentle pattern if someone throwns in a great boulder! *If the medicine is stronger than the disease, it will take over.* The original pattern of symptoms will only be removed permanently if the medicine is close enough in action to resonate with the original symptoms. If there is not enough resonance, the original stimulus remains untouched and unresolved. The medicine may be strong enough to supplant this with a new pattern, which may be more visible only because it is more dominant. In this case, when the vital force recovers from the action of the medicine, the original symptom pattern may reappear: the symptoms were suppressed rather than cured. The original disturbance was unresolved. See Figure 5.1.

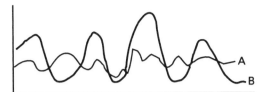

Fig. 5.1 If the above are ripples on a pond, B has much more energy than A, so A will disappear. B may create a greater disturbance with its own consequences which may prevent A from re-appearing. However, if the cause of A is not removed, it may simply re-appear when B is expended.

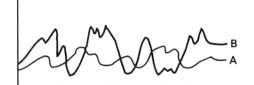

Fig. 5.2 In this pond, ripple A is so different from ripple B that it is possible that both will be altered – but the disturbance has been increased.

The new rhythm of the medicine may be so different as to exist side by side with the old rhythm, creating a new joint pattern! (Fig. 5.2) This may be possible when the areas affected by the medicine and by the disease are different, e.g. one affects the respiratory system and the other affects the digestive system. This situation is uncommon, as the disturbance and the medicine both affect the vital force, which reacts as a whole throughout each level of the organism.

The homoeopathic principle of cure is that one similar but stronger pattern is imposed over another, so that it takes over. Cure is aided by the fact that the duration of the medicine is limited, because it is potentized and kept to the minimum dose. Cure is indeed permanent if the remedy chosen is similar enough to include the total symptom picture and the exciting cause. If these are not covered, the disturbance is not truly solved because the predisposition or weakness remains and so there is a recurrence when vitality again drops or the exciting cause is met again.

ACTIVITY 3 If you are studying this course with a tutor, it may be useful to write a short essay on how the action of the medicine demonstrates the Law of Similars.

The Self-Limiting Action of a Medicine

In disease the medicine acts because it has a similar field of action to the disease (symptom picture), and resonates on these same areas of the vital force, encouraging the same action of the vital force which results in the outward movement of symptoms. This outward movement is clearly seen in acute diseases, and gives them their self-limiting nature. In acute disease we can see that the self-limiting nature arises from the ability of the vital force to reach the 'edge of the pond', i.e. acute diseases end either in death or elimination, as in the diarrhoea and vomit of cholera, or the spots of measles and chicken pox. A well prescribed remedy following the Laws of Cure will strengthen the outward movement of the symptoms, enhancing elimination. Thus there is a target to be achieved by the vital force, namely to push symptoms outwards as an elimination.

The remedy is self-limiting when prescribed in the single dose because the vital force is further disturbed by a substance whose nature so resembles the disease that it can take over. It is the ability of the remedy to obtain a stronger reaction from the vital force that enables the vital force to complete the action of elimination. It does this because the potency is selected to be stronger than the disease, so that it vibrates on a higher octave (see Lesson 8) where the nature of substance is less physical and there is less resistance to flow, i.e beyond the physiological level on to the dynamic plane. And because the dose is so minimal there is none left over to continue interference with the action of the vital force.

In acute illness we give a remedy and that is the end of the matter. The elimination is complete, and there are no repercussions or correspondence to other factors of health – it is a one-off situation. This does happen, especially in children, but it is a theoretical situation because the vital force is afflicted by miasms in such a way that its function is restricted.

In the constitutional picture there are weak organs and there are latent states where previous disease was unresolved – this is particularly so in the adult. The result is a lack of vitality and an inability to complete the work of resolution. Aided by a remedy the vital force may restore harmony to a greater degree, but a stronger stimulus may be required. This may be a further, higher dose of the same remedy, or another, different remedy, depending on the symptom picture. We can see that the idea is still to stimulate reaction from the vital force, but in this type of case the problem is to produce enough reaction at the acute level.

At the acute level, once you have thrown the stone into the pond the ripple pattern is created. The event is time-locked, it is past. The stone does not continue to disturb and once the reaction is complete the event is over.

ACTIVITY 4   Give three other examples to describe an event being time-locked and over.
Find two examples of illness, one which is acute and completely over when it is ended, and another which has repercussions that continue.

Susceptibility

Hahnemann and Kent use this term where Vithoulkas uses the word 'resonance'. In modern allopathic terminology it is used to describe the vitality of a patient, in that he or she is more or less susceptible (weakened) to the germs of a particular disease. In this last context it embraces the concept of vitality, or resistance to disease. However, in a homoeopathic context it is only used to imply resonance to the remedy or to the exciting cause.

Susceptibility to the remedy determines the degree of reaction to that remedy. One who is most susceptible to the remedy reacts easily to it, even in low potencies, whereas one who is least susceptible will barely react at all, and then perhaps only after repeat doses, as in the proving. The choice of potency will act to ameliorate or enforce the reaction to the remedy, so that one who is more susceptible may produce the same results from lower potencies than one who is less susceptible. Conversely, the least susceptible may not react at all to the higher potencies, which need even greater resonance as there is even more dilution in the higher potencies.

Susceptibility can be created by repetition of the dose. This is done in the proving. As soon as the vital force is touched it reacts, and that reaction immediately changes the situation. When disturbed, the vital force accommodates the disturbance and moves on.

If the disturbance is an ongoing factor in the environment, i.e. a maintaining cause, then part of the vital force's accommodation is to build a higher threshold of reaction. Thus the second dose must be a stronger stimulus to achieve impact. This is one reason why we go up in potency if we repeat a dose. After the first dose, susceptibility to that remedy or exciting cause may be less.

When another strong dose or repeated doses are given, the vital force is continually pulled back to the point it left, until the resonating parts of the vital force eventually react and become more sensitive to the stimulus because they are weakened. The process of cure is thus prolonged, because the vital force continues to be irritated without allowing the changes to take place which would lessen the organism's susceptibility. In the proving we stop taking the pills once the symptoms start to appear, and the vital force is left undisturbed. In order to resolve the disturbance the symptoms keep on appearing in the proving.

During treatment, this repetition of the dose can be dangerous because it creates greater weakness in areas already vulnerable. This is one of only two occasions when homoeopathy can be unsafe; the other is when too high a potency is used, when there is structural (pathological) change expressed in the symptoms. Here we also see why the homoeopath is cautious to accept that a remedy has created no change. If the remedy has struck so deep that symptoms have not yet appeared, then the vital force is reacting at a vulnerable level and has not yet been able to begin to correct the disturbance. To create further disturbance in such a case is undesirable.

When repeat doses are given you will often notice that there is no reaction at all until the dosing ceases. There may then be a very violent reaction. By continually stimulating the same point, an artificial disease will be created or the original disease may be worsened. The vital force is not free to act until the dosing ceases. The repeat stimulus may push the disturbance into a more chronic level if it is resonating on vulnerable weaknesses or, if this is not the case, deeper cure may result when the vital force gets to work with more energy. I do not advise repetition of the dose by the novice, as it is too easy to miss the point of change which indicates the enhanced movement outwards of the symptoms. This is part of the Law of Cure, which will be dealt with in the next lesson.

ACTIVITY 5   Write a paragraph in your own words to show what you understand by susceptibility.

The Speed of Action of a Medicine

The speed of reaction to the medicine depends on:

- The nature of the medicine;
- The vitality of the vital force;
- The nature of the exciting cause.

The Nature of the Medicine

Included in the character of a remedy is the speed with which it acts. Acute remedies such as Belladonna, Aconite and Apis Mellifica work very fast indeed and, as the name 'acute' signifies, they are of use in self-limiting situations, where they enhance the outward movement of the symptoms right to the edge of the pond. Other remedies have a slower reaction and are more suited to chronic disturbances. Examples of these might be Silica, Plumbum or Calcarea, to name some of the slowest. On studying a medicine it is necessary to know the pattern of symptoms it produces, and the depth and speed of action of which it is capable. In other words, what is expected when a remedy is given to a patient.

The strength of a remedy may be enhanced or lessened by the potency used. Higher potencies will act with greater speed than lower potencies, because the lower potencies are working nearer the physiological or physical level.

The Vitality of the Vital Force

A strong healthy vital force will react with speed, whereas a weakened vital force will act slowly because its areas of vulnerability are deep in organs and in metabolic processes. An indication of the vitality of the vital force may be gained by looking at the types and levels of symptoms being produced in the total symptom picture.

The Nature of the Exciting Cause

The exciting cause acts as a trigger. A patient may be susceptible to damp, and will react strongly and quickly if caught in a downpour, especially if the vital force is strong. In another patient there may not be a sudden response because the vital force is weaker, but because of the strength of the exciting cause, when the response comes it will be much deeper, as in pneumonia. Sometimes, even if the exciting cause is mild, as in an April shower, the weak vital force will still react on the organ level but this time it will produce bronchitis, which is of course serious enough, but less acute than pneumonia, so it is more chronic.

THE INTERPLAY OF THESE THREE FACTORS WILL DETERMINE WHAT WE MAY EXPECT FROM OUR TREATMENT.

Summary

The medicine stops acting when the vital force recovers from its impact. The medicine disturbs the vital force; it must do this with greater strength than the disease in order to be effective. The first action of the vital force under this greater burden is to sink a little (how much depends on the potency of the remedy and the vitality of the vital force). Then a stillness or quiet appears prior to adjusting, then the symptoms are thrown out with greater effort. The action of the remedy is thus ended, and the vital force is now reacting.

The vital force has corrected its susceptibility to the remedy and has moved on to clear up the mess. Further doses of the medicine will demand more reaction, will create more clutter to clear up, and cure is delayed. (This is why Hahnemann taught us the law of the minimum dose.)

If the medicine is continued it will disturb the vital force further, so that when the illness is removed further action of the medicine will become apparent. At first the symptoms may return, then increase in intensity, then other symptoms of the medicine will appear – the vital force now proves the remedy. If the medicine is further continued the vital force will be more and more directly afflicted. In some cases this might be wonderfully curative – it depends on the vitality of the vital force. If there is not enough vitality, the acute symptoms will enter a phase of chronic illness!

Disease acts by the same process. The vital force can easily adjust to some diseases, whereas in others the weaknesses that are affected are so fundamental that the vital force can not accommodate them, so it is severely weakened. Yet it still has to maintain life. It does this by allowing the disease process deeper into the body, localizing as far as possible, but prepared to sacrifice one part to save the whole. This is when organs are affected. You will study this later under the section on disease.

THE MEDICINE IS SELF-LIMITING BECAUSE ITS DOSAGE IS CONTROLLED, BECAUSE IT IS NOT REPEATED UNLESS THE SYMPTOMS, THE SITUATION, RETURN.

READINGS

Hahnemann S – *The organon*, paras 19–35, 52–70, 153–155, 157–160, 269–271
Kent J T – *Lectures on homoeopathic philosophy*, Chs 13, 14, 15
Vithoulkas G *The science of homoeopathy*, Ch. 11

REVISION

Put the following symptoms into hierarchies:

Case 1
Blowing noises in the air. Frightening dreams, especially late at night. Constipation plagued her. Menses are protracted and she is inclined to faint. She loses confidence easily, especially in new situations.

Case 2
The child has a sinking feeling in the abdomen, especially around mid-morning. He is not a lonely boy but spends much time on his own, engrossed in his pursuits. The skin is dry. The inside of his mouth is dry and tends to ulcers. He tends to have colds in winter, but feels generally worse in summer when the heat irritates him drastically.

Case 3
He has a scraping pain on the tibia that is worse at night. There is no history of injury. In the head there is a squeezing pain in the right temple which is worse in the morning and on moving. He is sullen and pessimistic, caring very little for anything since he lost his wife 3 years ago.

Case 4
She suffers from dizziness when she turns her head to either side. At night she sweats profusely in bed. She is slow by nature, thinks slowly, and cannot concentrate for long. When she eats she has difficulty passing food along the gullet. She has constipation also and urine stops and starts, refusing to flow continuously.

Case 5

The patient has pain in his joints which does not stay in one joint but wanders from joint to joint. It is particularly worse before rainy weather. He is afraid of thunderstorms. He is very sensitive to the cold and may be quite ill after alcohol. If exposed to the cold he often suffers from diarrhoea.

Case 6

He has ulcers on his tongue and very foul breath. Thick yellow catarrh comes up in strings that is difficult to draw forth. There is a great weight in the pit of his stomach, especially after drinking alcohol the night before. This does not happen too often as he tends to avoid the company of others.

Case 7

He is a tall thin individual, with a strange sensation of coldness, but only in small patches or spots. With this comes a sensation of numbness, but he feels as if something is crawling over his skin. He eats little as this leads to cramps in his abdomen. He develops diarrhoea after eating fruit. He is generally worse when the weather changes, and is restless.

Case 8

She has had painful periods for the last 2 years. She split up with her fiance then and has still not forgiven him for his unkindness. Thinking of this frequently prevents her sleeping at nights. She wakes in the morning with a thumping headache, especially before the menses. It is worse when she goes outside when it is sunny, despite the fact that the sun cheers her. She likes salty food and has much thirst, especially in the evenings.

Case 9

He has a polyp in the left nostril which first appeared when he was 14 years old. Otherwise he claims he is healthy, but does admit that he is easily exhausted and finds it difficult to concentrate on his studies. He is actually an anxious person who is easily excited, and although at first he appears full of enthusiasm he is easily discouraged. He strongly dislikes being on his own but is shy in company.

Case 10

She suffers severely from hiccups, which are worse when eating, drinking or talking. She says they are making her life a misery. She laughs when talking of this and fiddles with her fingers. She is a restless person. She is easily angered, then she becomes violent and wants to beat up others. She is suspicious that others deliberately goad her to weaken her. She is worse before menses, and in the morning after sleep.

SELF-ASSESSMENT QUESTIONS

There are some difficult philosophical concepts in this lesson, so study well the chapter in the textbooks to answer the questions below.

1) How do we know a medicine can affect the state of health?

2) What might happen in a proving if the prover was not healthy?

3) Explain how a medicine acts like a disease.

4) Name two factors that limit the action of a medicine in a patient.

5) What factors may influence susceptibility to the medicine?

6) Explain why it is unsafe to repeat a homoeopathic medicine.

7) Explain why a change in symptoms may only occur after the dosing of medicine ceases.

8) State three factors that affect the speed of action of a remedy. Which of these do you think is most important? State your reasons.

9) What happens to the vital force when we stimulate with medicine below the point of cure?

LESSON SIX

The Law of Cure

Headings: A Means of Assessing Treatment
The Organism as a Self-Perpetuating Mechanism
The Centrifugal Action of the Vital Force
Different Types of Change
The Law of Cure

Aims: By recognizing the direction of movement of the symptoms, by the end of this chapter you should be able to tell whether cure is taking place.

Objectives: To recognize the three types of change in symptoms;
To recognize that there are stages of degeneration in disease;
To recognize four directions in which symptoms change to produce cure.

A Means of Assessing Treatment

Without doubt, the Law of Cure is the most important practical dogma in the whole of homoeopathy. Whereas the similimum, the single remedy and the single dose give us the form or structure of homoeopathy, the Law of Cure is the working tool that enables us to evaluate precisely what effect our medicine is having on the patient. In more advanced work the Law of Cure will also give us a deeper insight into the disease process, as it becomes a means to measure how deeply the disturbance has penetrated.

It was Constantine Hering that formulated the Laws of Cure as we now understand them. They are drawn from many observations of the pattern of movement of the symptoms after treatment.

In paragraphs 12 and 17 of the *Organon*, Hahnemann tells us that cure is simply the removal of symptoms. He discovered that homoeopathic remedies are very effective at removing symptoms but, if after a period the patient develops a deeper group of symptoms, how can we explain that? Of course, this may be the result of a more intense or severe exciting cause. Hahnemann had a clear concept that each dose of medicine should free the vital force to greater health, and therefore this dilemma set him a puzzle which he answered with his theory of chronic diseases, or miasms.

If there are years between the two visits of the patient, feedback is inadequately slow. How can we ask someone to wait so long? In our geographically mobile society we may not see the patient in later years, so we do not know the long-term effects of our treatment. It therefore follows that, if we are to grow in our practical skills, we must have a more immediate and accurate measure of assessment of the treatment. This is provided by the Law of Cure.

The Organism as a Self-Perpetuating Mechanism

The theory of the Law of Cure makes several assumptions. The first and most far-reaching is that the organism is a self-perpetuating system with a self-regulatory mechanism – in other words, there is an intelligence which acts to perpetuate itself according to its own nature. Any movement away from that nature, for whatever reason, causes the intelligence to react to restore harmony and balance. Hahnemann calls this intelligence the vital force, and saw it as the coordinating intelligence of the whole (para 3).

The hidden process of the vital force is automatic and independent of any remedial treatment. The body is, at best, capable of curing itself. It is only when the vital force gets into trouble and cannot heal itself that it is the homoeopath's job to discover why, to identify exciting and maintaining causes, or any point of departure from harmony, and to remove blocks so the vital force can get on with its job. The purpose of treatment is to clear a way for the vital force to act. It is the organism itself, of its own nature, that is doing the healing. The homoeopath is simply removing the blocks to cure.

Of course homoeopathy is very different from other healing systems because it recognizes this action of the vital force, and (para 16) also recognizes that the medicine should be of the same nature and speak the same language in order to affect the action of the vital force, hence remedies are potentized because the vital force is non-material.

Having identified the blocks to cure, the second step in the healing process is to remove these, but to interfere only sufficiently to clear the block and to allow the vital force to act. In cure we see this as bringing the body to the point of change using the minimum dose, and then, following a policy of non intervention, we wait and watch.

The Centrifugal Action of the Vital Force

The phenomenon of the Law of Cure depends on the nature of the vital force to act in a rational manner. After treatment, the symptoms should change in an ordered manner, so that the last symptoms to appear go first. The last symptoms are more serious, as they show the deepest reaction of the vital force. If any vital organs are affected these are healed first. The movement is always from the centre outwards. There is a silent period, then it is as if the vital force has got the rhythm right and all the structural parts are aligned so the symptoms can proceed outwards, like the ripples in the pond, to spread the displaced energy and resolve the disturbance. A spinning top is a good image to have here too. The simple centrifugal pattern can also be observed in many areas of nature, from a giant star to the electrons in an atom.

In some of our remedies the simple centrifugal action is very clear, e.g. in the remedy Sulphuricum, which produces spots on the outside of the skin. The body is not quite spherical, though, and some parts are weaker than others, so other remedies show that specific areas of the body are selected. The vital force throws the disturbance as far out as possible. If it cannot reach the skin, either it does not have the energy to do this or the route is blocked by dysfunction in one or other system. A remedy must be chosen that deals with the cause of the disturbance – the exciting cause or maintaining cause – and then it must fit the same areas of weakness. Each homoeopathic remedy has an affinity with specific fields of activity, so the identification of levels of healing aids the choice of remedy.

- Some poisons deal with the digestive system, so vomit or diarrhoea expel the disturbance outwards through the normal excretory channels.
- The circulatory system touches every part of the body, so the heat of inflammation of fever indicates accelerated activity and presence of the blood to regulate the internal environment. Physically this may be seen as purifying fire burning out toxins.
- When the toxins cannot be destroyed in this way, they may be discharged as pus through the most convenient route, locally at the site of the wound, or systematically as it gathers at the lymph node – the tonsils in the healthy person, the synovial capsules or joints in a degenerate state. The mucus membrane may secrete catarrh in the upper respiratory system, or leucorrhoea in the urogenitary system.
- Some toxins have no route of exit so they are locked in as far out of harm's way as possible. An example of this is the insecticide DDT (dichlorodiphenyltri-chloroethane), which is not excreted but stored in the fatty tissue. Is it coincidence that fat is thrown to the outside of a centrifuge?

The signs and symptoms produced by the patient are a result of the healthy act of the vital force, externalizing the disease so we can use them to identify the seriousness of the disturbance. We can assess the potency of the remedy according to the elasticity or ability of the vital force to recoil or react, i.e. the speed with which the reaction comes. The type of symptom produced tells us the depth of the disturbance according to which level of defence or seriousness the disturbance has penetrated. The more vital the organ afflicted, the deeper the disturbance has penetrated and the more seriously ill the patient is. Thus we can use the symptom picture to assess how well the body is coping with the disturbance in terms of the Law of Cure. Examples are necessary.

If the heart is affected, the patient is much more seriously ill than a patient with eczema, because the heart is one of the most vital organs, affecting the integrity of the whole. If the patient with eczema develops heart problems then health is deteriorating. If the heart patient's problems disappear and an eczema develops on the surface, this patient is healthier, no matter how bad the eczema.

ACTIVITY 1

Play with a spinning top. Drop some objects on to its surface and see what happens to them. Interfere slightly and more greatly with its edges as it spins; what does it do? How much energy do you need to apply to correct these disturbances?

Different Types of Change

Sensation

If the symptoms remain at the level of sensation, the patient may not be so ill as another who has stones in the kidney or gallbladder. An example of symptoms at the level of sensation may be: I feel tired, I feel sick, my arms feel numb, there is a pain in my . . . . The sensations of dis-ease warn the patient that something is out of harmony. It is like hearing a funny noise in your car – stop now and something simple could be done. More sleep, less tobacco or fewer sweets, less exertion or more, are all simple remedies which could forestall worse problems.

Dysfunction

Using the car model further: we hear the noise but we drive on. The situation is not remedied but continues to deteriorate, so that jerking or chugging appears next. The function of the car is affected. In the body, this may be a change in rhythm so the body sweats more, or gets hot or cold, or develops constipation or diarrhoea. This change of rhythm or dysfunction may still be cured easily, although it is a more serious disturbance than a sensation. In dysfunction the parts compensate by either over- or under-functioning.

Structural change

Of course, if I drive the car on something will break. The car then seriously malfunctions. The body has reached the point of pathological change where the structure of the organs and/or tissues is damaged. This is a much deeper disturbance and will take longer to cure. It takes longer to develop disease in physical tissue, and it takes longer to regrow tissue than it does to change rhythm.

The progress of disease

If the symptoms are grouped into these three categories we may have an idea of how seriously ill the patient is, and what change can be expected following the Law of Cure, i.e. to move from pathology back to dysfunction and so to sensation. Pathological or structural change is the deepest of the three, and can be seen to be opposite to centrifugal action.

Pathological change internalizes and localizes the disturbance, so slowing it down into physical structure, where the vital force can drop an octave into less volatile physical matter, where at first the organism is less endangered. Were it to stay at the dysfunction level and more fever were needed, the temperature might go so high the organism would die. The vital force cannot allow this and must cope by finding another way of expressing the disorder, so to slow down the reaction the vital force allows it to move deeper, into slower-moving physical structure.

In looking at cases it will be noticed that each time the level of disease changes there is a silent period, or a lessening of the patient's distress, which may last for years. We should never be fooled into thinking the patient is then getting better. This is especially true of pathological change, because the living organism will accommodate some malfunctioning tissue until the proportion of this to the whole so increases that the organ cannot function properly. Only then does the whole feel the lack of that part. The liver is a good example of this. The liver will continue to function, or appear to function, although a large part of it is diseased. Of course pain etc. may come long before the final destruction of the organ, to warn that all is not well. This is the sensation level in the organ. Pain should stop us, warn us and give us more time to achieve a better balance

45

– unless the patient is unlucky enough to be prescribed pain killers; these will mask the problem until dysfunction appears.

ACTIVITY 2   Write down at least six examples of each of the three types of change.

The Law of Cure

The Law of Cure is very simple. In these days of gross pathology and suppression, however, it may require considerable skill in reading the relevance of symptoms and the level of disturbance, since there may be many organs and processes disturbed. Does any one of these really have priority, or does the job of the homoeopath remain to treat the whole? The answer is obviously that no cure is possible unless the whole is treated. A thorough analysis of the detailed disease process in any one patient is an advanced study. Here we will simplify the matter, but attempt to make it as practical as possible.

From Vital to Less Vital Organs

If there is anything wrong in a vital organ, no other symptom is put first, hence the homoeopathic aggravation in moving the symptoms outwards does not exacerbate the vital organ. Life is preserved, but a new set of symptoms may appear elsewhere. The patient may be aghast that she now has a sore throat, when before she only had menstrual cramps. Trained by allopaths, the patient separates the body into unconnected anatomical systems, and does not recognize that the new illness is only the steady process outwards of the old one. The homoeopathic remedy affects the vital force so that, in balancing from the centre, it withdraws the symptoms from the vital organ and places them one stage further out at a lower level of defence. The direction of movement is not arbitrary – there are definite relationships between organs, and it is often the case that the less vital organ previously showed some disturbance. Careful case-taking can trace the possible route outwards.

This law accounts for the lack of aggravation in emergency situations such as accidents. Where the vital force is healthy and there is no other disturbance, it starts its centrifugal action immediately, e.g. Arnica does not increase the clot in the stroke, neither does it increase the bleeding in a broken leg.

The chronically ill patient may be so exhausted that he or she cannot cope with the increased activity in the vital organ, and so may face prolonged aggravation because the vital force cannot resolve the situation or bring it to a crisis. Supporting the organ, 'organ therapy', or 'drainage' which increases the excretory processes, or 'diet' which cuts down any additions to the body's toxic load, or removing the 'maintaining causes', are all methods of treatment that recognize this first Law of Cure, that disease would not exist in the vital organ if it could fall further downwards into less vital organs. (I will have much more to say about the role of such therapies in managing the chronic case. Suffice to say here that any therapy should be linked to supporting the action of the vital force, which has an individual characteristic in each patient, therefore routine prescriptions must be frowned upon and we must put effort into studying the needs of each individual.)

From Within Outwards

This law shows a clear direction, and may account for the appearance of some new symptoms or the aggravation of other symptoms. As the disease switches from one anatomical system to another, it can be seen to externalize. Asthma again becomes eczema; this is a classic example of this law. Indeed, the homoeopath is happiest when skin eruptions follow remedies because this demonstrates the ability of the vital force to push the symptoms right to the surface. It shows vitality. Of course, from within outwards may also mean accelerated action in normal excretory processes, such as defecation, urination, menstruation and perspiration.

Eczema and psoriasis are perhaps exceptions to the rule here, as they are diseases of the skin as an organ rather than evidence of outer movement. They should be looked at carefully, because chronic illness on the whole indicates the inability of the vital force to resolve the issue, i.e. there are miasmic causes. Even so, you will recognize that it is progression to move from asthma to eczema, or from arthritis to psoriasis.

In acute disease, this second law is most usually seen in the increased rhythm of the normal organs of excretion; if these outlets are blocked, a secondary level capable of excretion may be formed by the lungs, or by the process of menstruation. After the administration of a remedy we may expect an increase in discharges, and these may be very foul indeed if there is a great deal of toxic waste. Leucorrhoea, catarrh, vomit, all represent the outward movement of symptoms.

If excretion or eruption on the surface of the body are prohibited, the healthy body may cope with the disturbance by producing a fever or inflammatory reaction, though this may have accompanied the eruption, as in measles or food poisoning. The involvement of the blood – fever or inflammation – is the usual speedy and acute reaction of the healthy body. A weaker reaction may be the involvement of the lymphatic system, as in a cold or tonsillitis. This is indicative of the suppuration process, where the mucus membranes produce catarrh. If there is no immediate external local cause, the first action of the body is to act generally, producing a fever. As the disease progresses it localizes and the whole process repeats itself on another level. Illness in an organ is first inflammation and pain on the surface of the organ, before any deeper structures or the entire function of the organ are disturbed. Structural change, ulceration locally, is the deepest level of change.

If we look at the development of lifeforms, this law can account for some interesting movement of symptoms.

These are the stages in development that recognize the appearance of

- an ectoderm
- an endoderm
- a mesoderm (Fig. 6.1).

Primitive animals and plants are first formed of a string of cells. Later this develops into a tube with an outer layer (the ectoderm) and an inner layer (endoderm) e.g. primitive worms. More evolved worms have a third layer of tissue that develops between the outer tube and the inner tube, which is called the mesoderm. In yet more evolved creatures such as humans, the ectoderm is the skin, so disease symptoms that can reach this level are healthier, or represent a more vital vital force, than in the case when symptoms develop on the endoderm – in humans this is the digestive tract, the urinary tract or the

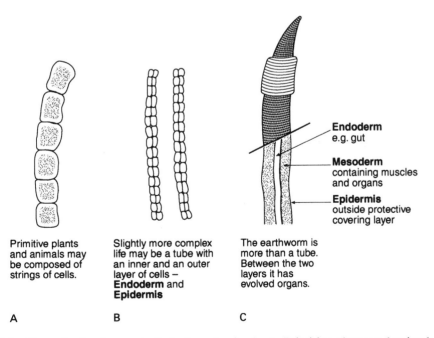

Endoderm
e.g. gut

Mesoderm
containing muscles
and organs

Epidermis
outside protective
covering layer

Primitive plants
and animals may
be composed of
strings of cells.

Slightly more complex
life may be a tube with
an inner and an outer
layer of cells –
Endoderm and
Epidermis

The earthworm is
more than a tube.
Between the two
layers it has
evolved organs.

A   B   C

Fig. 6.1 Stages in development of plants and animals. A. Primitive plants and animals may be composed of strings of cells. B. Slightly more complex life may be a tube with an inner and an outer layer of cells – endoderm and epidermis. C. The earthworm is more than a tube; between the two layers it has evolved organs.

respiratory system. The mesoderm of the human is affected by connective tissue disease, for example, which is more serious even than disease in the endoderm. If we remember that the mesoderm is the third tube, we can understand why disease there is deeper: it is more evolved or differentiated tissue.

From Above Downwards

This law may be discovered in the physical distribution of symptoms, e.g. eczema may increase as the disease is externalized, and should extend lower down the arm towards its extremity.

In some situations this law can be difficult to see. In the process of formation, the embryo twisted and contorted the body into some strange alignments. Symptoms that move further along the alimentary canal to the exit at the anus are moving from above downwards even though the move up the ascending colon and across the transverse colon precedes the movement down the descending colon. Symptoms that move up the respiratory system are heading towards the exterior and can be explained in terms of the second law, from within outwards, but the throat pain ascending to the ear is travelling up a drain from the ear and indicates a deepening of the situation. In the embryo the movement in the respiratory system is moving from the centre out to the edge of the egg!

Colds that move from the nose down to the throat and then to the chest are moving in towards the centre, towards more vital organs where they will affect the function of the body more deeply.

In Reverse Order of Appearance

The fourth law is concerned with the pattern of symptoms over time rather than space. It recognizes that the disease process proceeds in stages, with points along the route which have caused the vital force to deviate. The healthy vital force, after the disturbance, should be able to return to a state of balance – to the centre. When a block to cure is such that the vital force cannot return to the centre, then it endeavours to create a new harmony from a balancing point removed from the centre, i.e. a new centre of gravity. In homoeopathic terms we call this a miasm: the vital force has been damaged and there are weaknesses, since the new centre of gravity is not the most natural, so strain and stress are put on some organs. When it is disturbed in this new point of balance, the vital force will produce a new symptom picture based on its new weaknesses, i.e. during illness it will attempt to return to its new point of balance. Given extra energy (e.g. homoeopathic treatment) it will attempt to return to the natural centre; if it can do this it will return through each last balancing point, through each block in turn or each old pattern of symptoms, until it gets back to the centre again. We call this 'peeling back the layers of the onion', but it will be seen that the recurrence of the old symptom pictures take place in reverse order of appearance. The body goes back in time, releasing old trauma which it has never fully resolved. This process is well recognized in psychotherapy regarding mental trauma.

Of course there may not be enough energy to go right back to the centre, in which case the organism may stick at another symptom picture. Care must be taken not to represcribe when this process is taking place, because we do not always see what is going on inside the body and until it stops acting we do not know what point the vital force has reached, so *do not prescribe while the symptoms are still changing*.

We must be careful also to take thorough case notes, so that we can distinguish between this process of going back through old points and the changed symptom picture produced by the wrong remedy or potency. We will not go wrong if we remember that the body always acts rationally, so we should use the Law of Cure to thoroughly assess our treatment.

ACTIVITY 3 You will find it useful to write an account of an illness experienced by yourself or a member of your family, or a friend.

Note how the illness changes its representation at different times.

Note also how medication or treatment changes the symptoms.

Analyse what the vital force is doing in terms of the Law of Cure.

ACTIVITY 4

True or **False**?

A remedy has been given in the following examples. Do the changed patterns indicate the working of the Law of Cure?

	T	F
Swollen knee – swelling disappears after treatment and ankle swells.		_____
Sore throat with dryness becomes more painful 2 hours after the remedy, then a copious discharge begins.		_____
A burning throat disappears and after 6 hours an excruciating pain appears in the right ear.		_____
Cramps in the abdomen are increased 15 minutes after the remedy is given.	_____	
Chest pain follows abdominal pain and a loose bowel.		_____
Dry rough skin disappears and a cold with a runny nose follows.		_____
Extreme irritability follows depression.		_____
Stool changes from foul, bloody and very loose, to very loose stool with much mucus.		_____
Copious sweat appears after treatment for rheumatism.		_____
Two warts disappear from the finger of the left hand, to be replaced 1 month later by five verrucas on the left foot.		_____
A wart enlarges and starts to blacken following the remedy.		_____
On the day following the remedy, the patient urinates 15 times.		_____
The blueness of the varicose veins increases but the pain disappears.		_____
In the case of psoriasis with pus under the nails the fingernails fall off.		_____
Pain disappears from an arthritic knee after 12 hours, and it is less stiff in the morning.		_____
An itchy anus disappears after 3 hours; 2 days later the patient has three mouth ulcers.		_____
After the patient is given Pulsatilla, the head pain moves from the right temple to the left.		_____
Pain in the right ear follows administration of Belladonna for an inflamed throat.	_____	
Pain in sore wrist is now sharp, the swelling is down.		_____
Child who has been given Chamomilla eats pudding when told, with the rest of the family, the first meal after the remedy.		_____

ACTIVITY 5

What do you think happened next?

Write down some symptoms in no more than a few lines. Check your answers by looking at the direction of symptom movement.

1) The breast lump enlarges and throbbing pain appears the day after the remedy has been given.

2) Ten minutes after taking Belladonna the patient's temperature rises even further, from 37°C–39°C. Then after 20 minutes the patient begins to pour sweat, from the head in particular.

3) The asthmatic patient calms suddenly after the remedy, then falls asleep.

4) Much itching appears in the lower leg on the day following treatment by Carbo Vegetalis for constipation. The patient has a history of varicose veins.

READINGS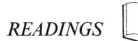

Hahnemann S *The organon*, Paras 157–160

SELF-ASSESSMENT QUESTIONS	Use the questions below to check your understanding of the text.

SELF-ASSESSMENT QUESTIONS

Use the questions below to check your understanding of the text.

1) The Law of Cure enables us to _____
   and _____
2) What is a 'point of change'?
3) Discuss how you see the vital force as acting rationally.
4) Give two examples of the centrifugal action of the vital force.
5) Name the three types of change in symptoms.
6) List the four Laws of Cure, and give an example of each.

The Homoeopathic Theory of Disease

Headings: Acute and Chronic Disease
            From Acute to Chronic Disease
            Miasms
            Acute Miasms
            Four Types of Acute Disease

Aim: By the end of this lesson you will know about the homoeopath's classification of disease.

Objectives: To understand the role of acute disease in cure;
            To understand how chronic disease arises;
            To understand the difference between four types of acute disease.

Acute and Chronic Disease

The homoeopath divides disease into three subcategories. Two of these are important and will be dealt with in this lesson in some detail. The third, pseudochronic, is not true disease, as the name indicates. Its existence depends on maintaining causes. When these are removed, pseudochronic disease is less of a problem.

Homoeopathic Classification of Disease		
Type	*Cause*	*Subtype*
Acute	Exciting	Epidemic Sporadic Endemic Contagious
Pseudochronic	Maintaining	
Chronic	Miasmic	Psoric: under-function Sycotic: over-function Syphilitic: mutated function

Acute Disease

In homoeopathic use *an acute illness is seen as short-lived and self-limiting, ending in either complete recovery or death.* This would agree with the allopathic use of the term to cover such illnesses as measles, typhoid, smallpox or chicken pox, but the homoeopath goes further in saying that *the acute illness, like symptoms, is part of the process of cure.*

As Part of the Process of Cure

When the acute illness is a simple cold, it can be seen clearly that the symptoms produced appear as an externalizing reaction to a disturbance of the vital force. Discharge and inflammation are common symptoms of a cold, and may arise after the patient has been exposed to cold dry winds, or received a soaking. Both of these causes are *exciting causes.*

An exciting cause disturbs the vital force, which of course responds by attempting to dissipate the disturbance.

The runny nose represents that Law of Cure that externalizes from *within outwards,* whereas the inflammatory process (fever and pain) represents the first dysfunctional level of disease. Pain in the throat is a sensation in the minor organs showing inflammation. In this case it is possible to say that the disease process has not penetrated

51

very deeply, irrespective of the intensity of the symptoms and despite the discomfort in an organ, because the discharge indicates the process of resolution.

As a Method of Creating More Health

The vital force also uses the acute phenomena of disease as a cleansing process. This ties in with the naturopathic ideal, and explains the symptoms that appear in a fast or other cleansing therapy, e.g. a sore head or a sudden diarrhoea, or even a sore throat. This shows *greater activity of the organism.*

The headache common at the start of a fast is a good example. When there is no food in the system to be metabolized, the liver has more time to do its other job as the major detoxifying organ of the body. Materials are then released from various locations where they were stored as harmlessly as possible. The toxins enter the blood on the way to the liver and kidneys, but this 'toxic' blood is also in contact with other parts, so headache and nausea and malaise may result. These symptoms pass as the process continues and the toxins are excreted. The severity of the symptoms depends on how much toxin was being transported, and this in turn may depend on how much energy is available to the cleansing process and just how seriously the body has been affected by stress, poor diet, bad habits etc. The less efficiently the body functions, the more debris that collects. When time allows, the healthy vital force will automatically start the cleansing process.

During inflammatory illness, the body automatically creates the space to detoxify when the patient loses his or her appetite and fasts naturally. In such illnesses the activities of the excretory processes are increased, even by sweating.

After a homoeopathic remedy it is common to see an acute illness appear. This may be a cold or a headache, or even diarrhoea. It is common after a homoeopathic remedy that the activity of the excretory organs should be increased.

As a Means of Lowering the Chronic Level

If the patient has a long-term problem, such as continually taking cold after the least exposure, then the homoeopath's assessment of the situation is that there is something wrong generally, i.e. that the vital force is chronically afflicted. Weakened and debilitated, the vital force will feebly attempt to resolve the situation by producing lots of little acute illnesses, but it does not have enough energy to produce a crisis in these to cure the chronic disease. The role of these acute illnesses is to prevent further degeneration of the chronic level. If more energy appears, (ie. after fasting, homoeopathic remedy, etc.) then the acute illness produced will be more severe, and more able to reach a crisis to create a better level of health.

Chronic Disease

This term is also used by the allopath, who applies it to cases of long-standing or recurrent illness such as arthritis, heart disease, asthma or eczema.

In homoeopathy the term chronic disease has a special place. It is used to represent lowered vitality, when the vital force is actually damaged and cannot restore harmony completely, although it will still do this as far as it is able.

Every one of us has chronic disease according to the homoeopath. Each has *an underlying pattern of weaknesses or predisposition that biases towards the exciting and maintaining causes to which we are most susceptible, and that condition the type of symptom we tend to produce.* This gives rise to the basic characteristics of an organism's health that the homoeopath labels a *constitution.*

If this were all it would be gruesome enough, but Hahnemann tells us that another characteristic of chronic disease is that it is a degenerative state. Because the vital force is damaged and has to settle at another centre of gravity, which puts stress on unfamiliar places not designed to bear such stress, there is continual and consistent wear and tear, which destroys health. Hahnemann says that the body afflicted with chronic disease degenerates until death. We can agree with this if we look at the common pattern of ill health in which a person gets weaker and more diseased as he or she gets older. The ageing process is an accepted fact.

ACTIVITY 1

List at least three of your predispositions.
What factors or exciting causes act upon these to produce acute illness?
Choosing one pattern of acute illness such as a cold or headache, list the symptoms and order their progress.

From Acute to Chronic Disease

The healthiest vital force will throw out disturbance rapidly, and even with force. The less healthy it is, the slower and less violent the reaction. The symptoms of the acute illness also vary in intensity, depending on the strength of the morbific agent to which the vital force reacts.

We can well conceive of a situation in which the vital force responds with violence. In one case it might be able to throw out the symptoms with great strength, but the temperature thus produced may be so high, or the diphtheria or pneumonia so intense, that the patient dies as a result. Not a pleasant situation, but remember that the acute illness is self-limiting, and there is either a full recovery or death. There is, however, an alternative.

The vital force can shift its expression of the disease so the process is slowed down. It is more chronic as it enters the deeper level, such as organs, where the physical structure slows down the disease. Thus a cold may enter the lungs, where it represents a more serious condition but may be less intense at first, thus giving more time for the vital force to preserve life.

The fact that the disease is more serious, though less violent or intense, is one of many apparent paradoxes we will come across in homoeopathy – a healthy person produces a cold with sneezing and temperature within hours of exposure, whereas a less healthy person takes several days of being below par before eventually the symptoms of flu appear. The flu affects more generally as it is the deeper disturbance, but it is the high fever of the cold which is most violent, and could even kill.

If the morbific agent is very great the vital force may be so affected that there is no possibility of expressing the disturbance. This situation is not unknown when psychological trauma is considered. The organism must hold the trauma until reaction is possible, but the very process of holding deflects its energy and introduces the resistance to flow that can then cause disease. The very process of holding the trauma handicaps the vital force's function in maintaining the integrity of the whole, and the pattern of constitutional weakness is produced. Such a state of the vital force is called a miasm.

It is of interest here that, *when the homoeopath strengthens the vital force to cope with the miasm, or any constitutional pattern, the process is reversed.* The slow, deeply seated action of the vital force is speeded up, the symptoms grow more intense, and the disease moves from the organs outwards. The acute stage is reintroduced.

ACTIVITY 2

You often hear that someone has 'never been well since' pneumonia or measles.
Do you know of such a case?
Compare the symptoms produced during the illness with those afterwards.
Is there a group of symptoms remaining after the illness?
In which organs or tissues are these produced?
Are these symptoms at an inflammatory or a suppurative level?
Did the symptoms of the actual illness contrast in any way to the normal expectations of such an illness?

Miasms

There are only three ways in which the vital force malfunctions. We have spoken of the vital force restoring harmony, and we have spoken of the action of a homoeopathic remedy in speeding up the action of the vital force. Using a further analogy with music, the vital force can be seen as a *rhythm*, which can be speeded up or slowed down or changed. Ortega in his book, *Notes on the Miasms* says only three changes to the vital force are possible. It can:

- Under-function
- Over-function
- Distort (mutate) function

These three are present as part of the disease process at all levels of severity. They can even be mixed up in one symptom picture at a different depth, or occur at different stages in the development of diseases.

The disease process involves first underfunction, then overfunction and finally distorted-function. For example, the first stage of the disease process is *inflammation* – a 'lack of' produces a need, so blood with its nutrients and heat is rushed to the spot to compensate. If this is not sufficient, the second stage, *suppuration*, occurs – excess often produces a discharge, e.g. the runny stage of a cold. Locally the third stage in a wound may be *ulceration* – healing is still not established and the tissue starts to change. Most mutations are of course destructive; very seldom is a mutation advantageous to the individual.

A disease pattern may enhance one or other of these stages, so bronchitis may represent the overfunction stage because it is most commonly accompanied by excess secretion, whereas asthma may represent the underfunction stage because it is usually an inability to breathe, following spasm in the bronchioles which causes them to close. However, some bronchitic illnesses are very dry (underfunction) and some asthmas are precipitated by excessive mucus in the lungs (overfunction). Pneumonia can be seen to contain all three stages, since it begins with inflammation, then often produces copious expectoration and, if allowed to progress far enough, enters the hepatization stage when the lung tissue changes structure. Depending on the individual constitution, one particular stage may be most important in any one patient. In each case of pneumonia, the full symptom picture of the required remedy will reflect this pattern.

Any one patient may have underfunction, overfunction and distorted function present at different levels, e.g. very dry skin, copious catarrh from the mucous membranes, especially severe leucorrhoea and, on the mind level, suffer severe delusions which are aberrations of consciousness. Again, one level may be more important than another. In general, underfunction is least serious because it is slower, and distorted function is the most serious because it is destructive, but of course it depends on the level: asthma (underfunction) is more serious than ulcers on the tonsils (distorted function).

Note that I have not yet used the word miasm to cover the patterns of expression of symptoms. The homoeopath uses that word to apply to the overall bias of the constitution, when a person is shy and lacking in confidence, with a tendency toward illnesses such as constipation and asthma, then he or she is said to *underfunction* constitutionally. Similarly, he or she may be described as *overfunctioning* if he or she is possessive, over-emotional (perhaps weepy or touchy) and inclined to produce illnesses such as excessive catarrh, sinusitis, tonsillitis, gonorrhoea. The patient with *distorted function* may be violent and angry, or so greatly introspected as to be morbid, and may produce illnesses such as gastric ulcers, acrid excoriating discharges or sweat, or Crohn's disease.

It was Hahnemann who first discovered these patterns. He found that homoeopathic treatment produced only temporary relief, and perhaps even long-term upset, if it did not reach deep enough to the source of the disturbance. Such deep treatment is very skilled indeed, and will be dealt with elsewhere. It is important to know the patterns at this stage, and to know that Hahnemann gave them the names we still commonly use, namely:

- Psora: underfunction
- Sycosis: overfunction
- Syphilis: distorted function.

Psora he saw as the origin of all disease, arising from the suppression of skin problems. He particularly singled out the suppression of the itch of scabies, and saw leprosy at the

54

extreme end of the psoric line of disease. The other two names he gave because through his experience he saw the patterns arising most commonly after the suppressive treatment of gonorrhoea (old name sycosis) and syphilis. Personally, I feel the miasms do not arise so much from these circumstances today, in Britain at least, so the names tend to lead to confusion. I also cringe when students start delving into the patient's past or even his/her parents past to uncover the history of gonorrhoea or syphilis that must be there because the patient is obviously sycotic or syphilitic. It offends more than little old ladies!

The importance of miasms at this stage in the course is not so much for prescribing, since we are still far from that point, but to aid the study of the patient's symptoms and the disease process, and also to enable better understanding of the essence of homoeopathic remedies. *The pattern of symptoms produced by a remedy will fall into one of these categories in the main, so we can talk of a sycotic or a syphilitic remedy.* We will also learn much more about the remedy through studying the path by which it reaches this main phase, i.e. the pattern of the disease produced by the remedy in its proving.

ACTIVITY 3 List ten symptoms in each of the three categories, to show under-, over- and distorted function.

Acute Miasms

You may come across this term in some books, so a few words here are appropriate.

An acute miasm occurs once in a lifetime. Diseases such as measles, chicken pox, mumps, rubella, whooping cough, diphtheria, polio, smallpox, etc. are examples. They are almost all childhood illnesses, and that is the clue to their role. An acute miasm is as it says, an acute expression of the underlying miasm. The vital force of the child is much stronger than that of an adult, so it can attempt to throw out, through an acute illness, what an adult could not. Through the childhood illnesses, the stronger vital force of the child attempts to unburden some of the miasmic load it has inherited. Later on, polluted and devitalized by the environment, and by stress and bad habits, it cannot do this, or if it does, the childhood diseases are often much more severe in the adult.

So, an acute miasm is a special kind of acute disease that strikes deep enough to change the constitution, and this is why the homoeopath does not believe in suppressing diseases such as mumps, measles, chicken pox, rubella, etc.

Four Types of Acute Disease

Before we leave this section on disease, it is necessary to look at four other labels – sporadic, epidemic, endemic and contagious (infectious). Again, the terms are commonly used by the doctor and since germs are seen as the main causative factors they are often used to challenge the homoeopathic theory of disease. If there is an epidemic of flu etc. around, how can the homoeopath explain why so many 'catch' it if it is not the germs that are passed on? Pasteur gave the clue when he said that it was the soil that enabled the germs to grow. We will learn more if we ask *who* catches the disease, and *what* is it they catch?

Epidemic

Not everyone catches the flu, and even those who do produce an individual variation of it. The next time there is a flu epidemic, take out your notebook and study the symptom picture. Homoeopathy is based on precise observation and collection of data. Examine the symptoms of those who catch the flu and you will find, without exception, that each had a *lowered vitality*, and particular reasons for that lowered vitality. But this is not enough. There are yet others who do not catch flu, and yet they too may have lowered vitality. Look again at those who catch flu, and you will find that they share a *predisposition* that makes them more inclined to catch flu – they are susceptible to similar exciting causes; they have weak lungs, or a tendency to sore throats or swollen tonsils, or gastric problems in some cases, or they may all have a weakness to a particularly cold dry spell that has arrived, or Christmas has just passed and the mortgage rates have risen and worry is crippling them! People react to factors in their environment, a fact maybe enhanced by increased media consciousness: illness as a group phenomenon.

Sporadic

Sporadic disease is more easily explained homoeopathically since it isolates certain individuals or groups seemingly at random. The above arguments apply – that a group or an individual succumbs because of susceptibility to certain exciting causes and lowered vitality, plus the predisposition to produce a relatively similar group of symptoms. We need only study the pattern of the disease and the nature of the group to recognize those at risk.

A sporadic disease is either too weak to seek out and affect the majority, or, more likely, it is unusual and so does not resonate with the majority.

Endemic

Endemic disease is associated with a specific place. Malaria is a good example of this. It is associated with swamps and the kind of temperatures that allow mosquitoes to breed. The environment is hostile to humans, and is it not strange that we accept that plants and animals need an optimum environment to foster healthy growth, yet deny the same for humans? Yet not all individuals develop malaria just by being in the vicinity of swamps, or after being bitten by an infected mosquito, although most do if continually exposed. The exciting cause may be virulent, or continual exposure may wear down the vitality, but the predisposition must also be there and it is important to recognize this in order to strengthen the vital force through homoeopathic treatment.

Contagious

Hahnemann speaks of contagious disease as an epidemic that prevails among densely congregated masses of human beings. The exciting cause or morbific agent is virulent, but it would have no effect if the predisposing weakness of the vital force were not present in each person afflicted. Vitality also plays a part, but the nature of the contagious disease, like the epidemic, is that it is so resonant to the vital force of many individuals. Today we would call this class 'infectious'. There is an ease with which the condition seems to pass from one individual to another. Hysteria, laughter, sympathy, gloom, itch are examples. Is it a bug that is passed? Perhaps so. Some catchy tunes are so virulent that it is impossible not to tap the feet, or to go around for days afterwards humming it at every odd moment. What is the mechanism for transference?

The orthodox practitioner will say the cause is germs. So, you might ask, what is wrong with this? There are many other parts of the equation to balance up. The facts show that many diseases disappeared when hygiene was introduced – the enteric diseases disappeared rapidly from Britain after the Public Health Acts of 1875, without a vaccination programme or new drugs. Many more diseases are now on the increase as environmental factors, poor housing and diet, industrial pollution and stress, bad habits such as lack of exercise, are ignored. Others have disappeared as certain aspects of the environment and diet have improved. While the public waits for the doctor to conquer another virus, the 'soil' is seriously neglected. As doctors have concentrated on eliminating acute disease, chronic disease has rapidly increased, so that even children have chronic degenerative diseases today.

If you are going to be a good homoeopath you must learn to think for youself and to question everything. Your assessment of the case must be based on sound logic and observation. In this last section I have leaned very heavily to one side so that, after weighing the current bias, you can achieve a more balanced approach and keep an open mind. Science should have no sacred cows, and no theory is truth.

ACTIVITY 4 Find an example of each of the four types of acute disease and describe the resulting symptom picture.

READINGS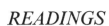

Hahnemann S *The organon*, paras 46–52, 70–104, 146–149
Kent J T *Lectures on homoeopathic philosophy*, Chs 7, 17. Review 9, 11 & 12
Vithoulkas G *The science of homoeopathy*, Chs 8 & 9. Review 7

FURTHER READING

Shepherd D *1967 Homoeopathy in Epidemic Diseases*. Health Science Press, London

---

SELF-ASSESSMENT QUESTIONS

Use these to assess your understanding of the text.

1) What is the difference between the homoeopath's and the allopath's use of the terms acute and chronic?

2) How can an acute illness be seen as creating better health?

3) What is the advantage of chronic disease over acute disease?

4) Is there a problem when chronic disease is cured?

5) List three ways in which the vital force can be changed.

6) If measles is an acute miasm of psora, how would you relate mumps and chicken pox to the miasms?

7) Which three factors affect the vital force's susceptibility to disease?

8) How does the role of these factors differ in epidemic, sporadic, endemic and contagious disease?

9) Discuss how a negative state can predispose to disease.

LESSON EIGHT

Selecting a Potency

Headings: Introduction
A Model of Potency Action Using Water
Light on a Few Questions
A Model of Potency Action Using Sound Waves
Some Questions Answered
How Do We Select the Potency Needed?
The Collective Single Dose, the Ascending Collective Dose and the Split Dose

Aims: This lesson will show that potency is an energy, and that this has a relationship to the type of symptom produced by the patient.

Objectives: To understand how potency is an energy;
To understand how the energy of the organism is represented by the level of symptom produced;
To choose a potency according to the level of energy or symptom produced by the organism.

Introduction

Despite homoeopathy's long history, the subject of potency selection is still a vague and arbitrary area which is seldom clearly understood. Kent has said that 'The selection of the best potency is a matter of experience and observation and not as yet a matter of law'. In the past, homoeopaths have divided into camps depending on whether high or low potencies were used; the antagonism between these camps was often violent, highlighting the fact that potency is frequently a matter of faith. The very fact that this question 'which potency?' keeps recurring shows a failure to provide a rational explanation to guide students of homoeopathy. What follows may thus be seen by some as controversy, but by applying the laws of science regarding energy, and by looking at the human being as a dynamic organism, I hope to take much of the mythology out of potency selection.

The remedy is potentized because Hahnemann discovered that the larger the crude chemical dose, the longer the patient takes to recover because the organism is more greatly affected by the medicine. In the case of crude chemicals this may even prolong the illness beyond its natural course, because the organism may need to deal with an excess of an alien substance before it can start the process of cure. Indeed, clearing debris from the body may be the first step of cure.

The potentized remedy initially increases the symptoms – the process of aggravation – because it increases the activity of the vital force. Because the dose is so minuscule, its action is merely to stimulate reaction. It does not clog up the body, so the potentized remedy can resolve the disturbance in a much shorter time period than the crude dose.

Why is the illness relieved more speedily by higher potencies? An easy answer is that the homoeopathic remedy is accurately modified for resonance with the vital force, and so its effect is more powerful. Let us try and simplify this a little by looking at models.

A Model of Potency Action Using Water

If I throw a stone into a pool of water, the disturbance will appear as a pattern of ripples moving outwards from the centre, just like the action of the vital force (Fig. 8.1). The pattern will vary according to the shape and size of the stimulus. The shape of the stone is analogous to the symptom picture of the remedy. Also, the size of the stimulus corresponds to the amount of energy mass or dose of the remedy. A big boulder will cause a greater disturbance than a little pebble, and the pattern the big boulder makes will take much longer to disappear, whereas the pattern made by a little pebble will quickly resolve itself (Fig. 8.2). Thus the more gross the dose the greater the disturbance, and the longer this disturbance is prolonged. This is true if only the size is different, i.e. the shapes of the stimuli are similar.

This model shows that the crude dose can create more disturbance, and it throws some light on a few questions.

Light on a Few Questions

The Effect of Multiple Crude Doses

Allopathy uses massive amounts of crude chemical drugs in multiple doses. These are like big boulders, and it should be noted that they create a pattern which is opposite to the pattern already created by the reaction of the vital force to the disturbance. The allopath standing on the side of the pool throws in so many boulders, creating such a disturbance, that the original ripple pattern is obliterated, and to make sure that the original ripples do not reappear the medicine is repeated frequently (Fig. 8.3).

Note that a new and totally different disease has now been introduced if the symptom picture of the medicine differs from that of the original disease, and note that the original pattern will return when the medicine is ceased if the cause of the disturbance remains.

Palliation and Suppression

It is possible to choose a medicine with a similar enough pattern to the original as to merge with it, so that the original is obscured or camouflaged without being resolved. This may happen because one pattern fits inside the other, uniting with it to give the appearance of a third pattern (Fig. 8.4). This is palliation, when the original symptoms appear to have receded in intensity. The intensity will return when the medicine stops.

If the homoeopath continues to repeat this stimulus, it is possible to prolong the camouflage pattern without resolving the original, which remains because the cause remains. When the symptoms disappear to find another outlet, usually at a deeper level, the homoeopath calls this suppression. Often there is a silent period between the disappearance and the reappearance at a deeper level. Palliation and suppression appear to happen more easily with homoeopathy because we use single remedies, and because the remedies are potentized to a pure level of vibration.

More Reaction with Low Potencies

Of course, there is a situation where the camouflage pattern is similar enough to the original to resolve it. The homoeopathic remedy is the similimum not the same. In low

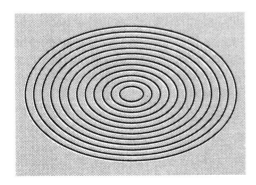

Fig. 8.1 Ripples spread outwards from the centre.

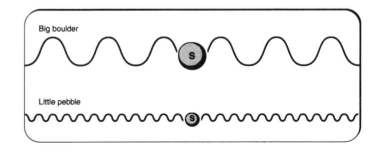

Fig. 8.2 As the stimulus is dropped into the pool a ripple pattern appears depending on the shape of the stimulus, the size and depth of the pool, and the speed and direction of the current. The intensity of the disturbance depends on the size of the stimulus: the greater the mass, the more water will be displaced and so it will take the ripple pattern longer to disappear.

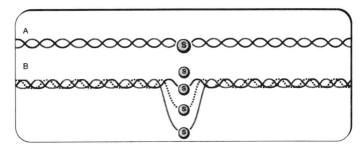

Fig. 8.3 A. When the second stimulus is added the phasing may not exactly match that of the first, so a greater disturbance appears and takes longer to resolve. B. Many more stimuli are added, and so even if the shape and size are constant the phasing is absent and such a disturbance is created that the original pattern is lost out of sight.

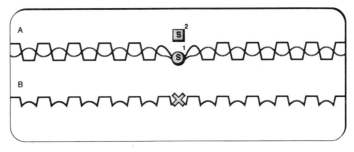

Fig. 8.4 A. S1 and S2 are different in shape and so may produce different wave patterns. B. The shape of the ripple pattern that may appear on the surface. This resembles neither of the first two, and so creates a third but artificial pattern.

potencies remedies are like pyramids – that which is most individual is at the apex of the pyramid, and what is most common is at the base. Since each of us has two arms and legs and a whole range of organs that function similarly, there is a considerable overlap at the base of the pyramids. Any one physiological malfunction has a limited variety of manifestations, so that almost any of the innumerable remedies that affect that manifestation may also affect the specific malfunction. On the physiological level, i.e. the level of common symptoms, there may be more than one homoeopathic remedy capable of curative action. This is invaluable in a first-aid situation, where the number of available remedies is limited (Fig. 8.5).

The Single Dose

It should be clear that the repetition of the dose is unnecessary if the chosen remedy is similar enough in shape (symptom picture) and intensity to the original stimulus. The idea is to produce an artificial disease (remedy) which has a symptom picture similar to the natural disease, so that it can interact with it. Just enough energy is introduced to stimulate and speed up the movement of the waves. Like a musical note, the two will

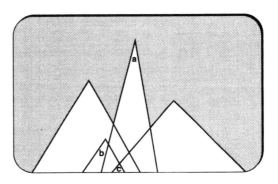

Fig. 8.5 At point (a) only one remedy covers the symptom picture; at point (b) two remedies cover the symptom picture in part; at point (c) four remedies cover a section of the symptom picture.

become one and the outward movement of the vital force will be enhanced. This is the curative act which resolves the situation. Another stimulus will prolong the disturbance pattern as it will confuse the vital force by putting all out of phase (Fig. 8.6).

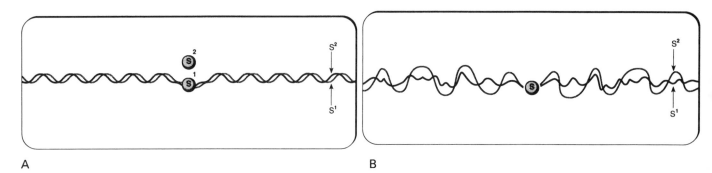

A   B

Fig. 8.6 A. S2 creates a second ripple pattern which is only slightly out of phase with S1, and therefore it joins with S1, perhaps moving faster to resolve the situation and restore calm. B. S2 is not the same as S1, but because its peaks and troughs coincide with some of those of S1 it can strike harmonies that interact with S1 to resolve the situation.

ACTIVITY 1   Visit a local stretch of water and experiment with a few stones, or watch the whirls in your bath water.
This time you should have a deeper understanding of the movement.
More questions will arise.

A Model of Potency Action Using Sound Waves

The water model used above is a simple mechanical one, on the horizontal plane. There are other concepts it cannot explain.

If we stimulate a time–space pattern with the similimum, three things may happen:

- If the stimulus is too small in energy the ripple pattern will scarcely be affected – this is the pebble, similar in shape but small in size (Fig. 8.7).
- If the stimulus is too great in energy the ripple pattern will be greatly increased and prolonged – this is the boulder, similar in shape but great in size (Fig. 8.8).
- It is the stimulus that has the same intensity as the cause which will most quickly resolve the disturbance – this is the optimum dose (Fig. 8.9).

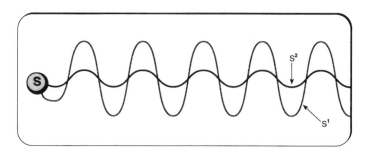

Fig. 8.7 The frequency of the wave pattern is similar in S1 and S2, but S2 does not reach the intensity of S1. S1 and S2 are the same shape but not the same size. S2 will have some effect on S1 because of its similarity, but this may be limited. If S1 is the symptom picture produced by the disease, then S2, the remedy, cannot cure unless its intensity is increased.

The dilemma that must now be considered arises from the fact that the effectiveness of a homoeopathic remedy increases with 'potency', so that the most dilute remedies are in fact the most powerful. From the above we would expect the greater mass to displace the greater volume of water, so creating the greatest disturbance, but in homoeopathy it is the smaller that creates the greater disturbance. It is paradoxical that the highest potency may be a big boulder disguised as a little pebble. How can this be?

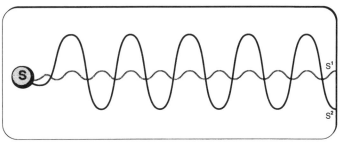

Fig. 8.8 The second stimulus greatly enhances the disturbance and deepens it, but being much greater than S1, the disease, takes over from it completely and must therefore be resolved itself if the difference is too great. Hahnemann explains that it is necessary for the remedy to create an artificial disease to take over from the natural disease in order to dispose of the natural disease.

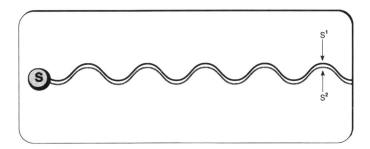

Fig. 8.9 The stimulus most similar in shape (symptom picture) and size (potency/strength) to the original disease stimulus resolves the situation most quickly.

A Change in Octave

Hahnemann told us that the greater effect from higher potencies comes because the potentization process puts the medicine on the 'dynamic plane'. In today's language we would say that we have released the energy from the material substance of the remedy. To grasp the paradox, we must change the model from wave patterns in water to sound waves that disturb the air. Although the mechanical motion is the same, although in a different medium, we recognize levels of energy in sound waves which are labelled octaves. We can then recognize that the *potentization process is a change in octave*, not in size. When the remedy is potentized it may become smaller in size, but it is also refined to a level of energy that is more volatile and reactive.

Life Energy Dances Faster or Slower

In the potentization process the nature of the remedy is not changed, except that the homoeopath recognizes that the more potentized or diluted the remedy, the more it is inclined to affect the more refined and non-physical parts of the human, the mental and emotional symptoms. The life with which we are imbued is a form of energy which reacts with energy, as in a dance. This gives us very different repercussions from the last model.

The remedy produced by the potentization process still acts to harmonize with the ripple pattern, but its levels of action are now increased as the potency varies (Fig. 8.10). The mechanism of resolving the disturbance is the same as explained above, but now we can add that, depending on the octave, the speed of dissolution may be faster or slower. Physical disturbance is slower to resolve as the dance of the atom is slower in the solid physical form, so lower slower potencies are to be thought of. The speed of thought is probably faster than the speed of light, and we know the mind is the greatest healer as well as the greatest destructive force. By giving the remedy at the level of mind, we can resolve the disturbance more speedily and more safely. This is the key behind Kent's use of high potencies: he was aiming at gentle cure on the level of the mind, where energy flowed faster and with less resistance.

How Potency Resonates

As the octave is increased, so the speed of vibration increases the energy. At low vibrations sound is felt physically, whereas at higher vibrations it may be described as piercing, and at even higher vibrations, as in a dog whistle, there is no longer resonance with the human ear. Thus potencies affect the organism differently.

63

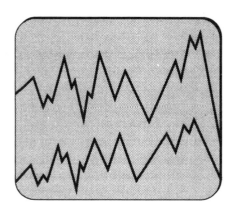

Fig. 8.10 The shape of the energy wave is the same but the energy level is different. However there is still a correspondence between the two notes, just as the C of one scale is related to the C of another.

Lower potencies may only affect the physical level, and higher potencies may be needed to affect the mental level. However, potencies are not confined to one level but will harmonize with symptoms on intervening levels. All levels of the organism are interconnected by various relationships, associations and cause and effect, and thus after treatment the patient may frequently uncover the feelings (anger, grief, indignation etc.) that have been transmuted into physical illness.

The musical note is not a passive isolate. It springs into existence when a tuning fork sounds the same note. A glass vibrates in frequency when it hears its note. A reciprocal note on the next octave will call the note into existence. The note will call forth harmony, harmonious notes and overtones (notes on higher octaves). Two notes of the same frequency blend into one. The life of the musical note is thus quite dynamic. The human organism has many levels of reaction – physical, emotional, mental and spiritual – and these interact with potency in predictable ways.

Some Questions Answered

Non-reaction to a High Potency

If a patient drops a brick on his toe the causation is external and physical, acting on a particular and only possibly affecting the general level. One might assume the patient needs a 6th or a 30th potency of Arnica, but all we have is a 50M. Will it act? The resonant remedy will act in all cases, irrespective of potency, because it can build a harmonic bridge, but the gap here is enormous and the remedy's ability to act may depend on the vitality of the vital force. A 50M may not be able to resonate on the physical level in some patients: the leap in energy levels may be too great to build a harmonic bridge, just as the coil in the car will produce a greater voltage only if the distance between the two 'wires' is within a certain range.

Non-reaction to Low Potencies

Similarly, if the cause is on the mental level a low potency may not produce enough energy to build a harmonic bridge to that level. The action of a homoeopathic remedy depends on resonance, which is the similarity of the symptom picture and the energy represented by potency. Repetition of the low potency, like Chinese torture, may create the harmonic bridge that will eventually sound the note on the higher potency level, which can then neutralize the cause (Fig. 8.11).

The Appearance of Proving Symptoms

What happens when the potency is too high? It may be like using a sledgehammer to crack a nut. Would you use a 10M potency to cure a headache? The field of action of a remedy can be described as being like a cone or a pyramid. A headache as a physical symptom will be found low down at the base of the pyramid; the 10M potencies will be found much nearer the apex of the pyramid. But if there is no disturbance above the physical level then we will create disturbance there if we use a 10M potency (see Fig. 8.11).

Other symptoms will appear which will be found to be of a proving nature, or if the remedy is sufficiently similar to the constitutional remedy of the patient it may simply use the excess energy to cure a few other problems the patient was unaware of, especially

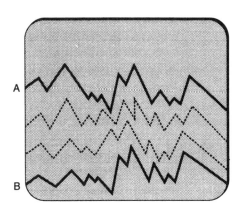

Fig. 8.11 B is the disturbance pattern of the disease; A is the wave pattern of the remedy. If the two have a harmonic relationship there may be other notes sounded in between, other symptoms appear during cure, or other symptoms cured during the action of the remedy.

if these are on the mental and emotional level. Proving symptoms will pass away quite quickly, depending on the vitality of the vital force and its susceptibility to the actual remedy given.

The Optimum Dose

It should be clear from what has gone before that the potency should not be too high or too low. There is an optimum dose which will resolve the symptom picture with least aggravation and few proving symptoms. There is considerable skill in choosing this, because we have no means of accurately measuring the amount of energy needed to resolve the disturbance, i.e. to measure the remedial action of the organism. There is a yardstick which will be discussed in the next section.

ACTIVITY 2

For this you will need a musical instrument, preferably a piano, and I would like you to listen to:

Some chords and notes played in harmony;
Some notes played in different octaves;
The effect of two notes played close together;
The disharmony of notes slightly further apart.

How Do We Select the Potency Needed?

We can now account for the prolonged aggravation of the lower potencies, over-reaction and non-reaction to higher potencies, the need to repeat lower potencies sometimes, the detrimental effect of too much repetition, and we have emphasized the need to select the optimum potency for the fastest safest resolution of the disturbance. The most important question is, of course, how do we recognize the potency needed?

Kent and others established a harmonic series of potencies which we still use: the 6th, 30th, 200th, 1M, 10M, 50M and CM. From them we inherited the yardstick that:

- Below 30 was for physical disturbance;
- 200 was for emotional disturbance;
- 1M and over was for disturbance on the mental plane.

My first comment on this is that it is only a yardstick. The potency chosen depends on the reactivity of the vital force and may change with the choice of remedy, as each has his or her own scale of action (see Fig. 8.10).

Some remedies are better in certain potencies and less effective in others. This may relate to Paul Callinan's work in Australia. By freezing remedies at −200°C he discovered that each remedy produced its own distinct pattern of crystals, like a snowflake, and whereas the pattern became clearer as the potency increased it also fluctuated, sharper and less distinct, then sharper again as the potency was raised. Thus the 6X was sharp, the 9X indistinct, and the 12X sharper again and more precise in definition than the 6X. He confirmed that the series of fluctuations coincided with the main potencies used today 6, 30, etc. However, at the time of writing he still had more work to do on the higher potencies. It is useful to identify the potencies at which the different remedies work best. This may be achieved by a deeper study of Materia Medica, and especially of the symptoms produced by each potency in the proving.

Kent's yardstick is useful, but crude as it stands. Adding Hering's Law of Cure will create a diagnostic tool that is more refined.

Physical Symptoms First: 6th Potency

The healthy vital force first produces physical symptoms, since it has the ability to reach right to the edge of the pond. These physical symptoms usually occur on the level of sensation or local inflammation, e.g. headache. There may be local suppuration in a cut, or an increased rhythm in the normal organs of excretion (bladder, bowels, sweat) after food poisoning or travel sickness. A 6th potency is sufficient to just touch the vital force, causing a physiological response. Where this reaction is stronger, as in acute remedies such as Aconite and Belladonna, a 30th potency may be required.

The General Level and Intense Physical Level: 30th Potency

If the reaction of the vital force is stronger, producing generalized fever, then the 30th potency may be necessary rather than repeated doses of the 6th potency; or it may be that the vitality was weakened, or the exciting cause was stronger so the disturbance penetrated deeper, giving rise to influenza rather than just a local cold. Influenza involves sensation on the general level (aches and pains all over) and a change of rhythm at the general level (fever, chill, sweat). Sometimes the local inflammation may be so intense as to require the 30th potency, especially if there are further developments on the general level such as fever, diarrhoea or nausea, or even if suppuration sets in. The 30th potency may also be given to mild emotional states, such as examination nerves or childhood trauma.

Emotional Turmoil and Violent Acutes: 200th Potency

When the vital force produces more violent acutes, such as dysentery and typhoid, or even in severe cases of influenza, inflammation may be life-threatening on the general level, as in fever, or the change in the rhythm of the excretory organs may be violent, and again possibly life-threatening. The 200th potency covers the case when the physical symptoms manifest with such violence – even a 1M potency may be considered.

The turmoil of the 200th potency is usually the province of emotional energy. Indeed, such an acute condition may arise from strong emotions and so upset the economy of the body that the patient cannot sleep, but turns and tosses, has a gnawing ache in the stomach yet a revulsion for food, or may have severe diarrhoea. If the cause is severe enough, again one would consider the 1M potency. Emotional remedies such as Ignatia are often better given in a 1M potency.

The Level of Temperament and Constitutional Treatment: 1M or 10M Potency

The 1M and 10M potency level is usually applied to constitutional treatment, especially where there are no pathological problems or structural change in any of the organs. At this level of stimulation we can reach the cause on the higher octave, and so change all the octaves below. At this potency level we are treating the symptoms at the apex of the pyramid, where the symptoms are most individualized. Strong resonance (accuracy in remedy selection) is necessary for reaction.

The Lower the Vitality, the Lower the Potency

When the outwards movement of the vital force is prevented – because it has insufficient vitality to reform the situation, or because the process of resolution would endanger the integrity of the whole, or because allopathic treatment has suppressed the vital force – the symptoms become more serious and the process described above is reversed, localizing in organs, first as inflammation and change of rhythm, and eventually as structural change. The closer the organism approaches structural change the lower the potency that is used. At this level the amount of action is limited and very slow, so the 6th potency is used. Before this stage is reached there is first the inflammation, and perhaps discharge, e.g. pneumonia or bronchitis, for which we might use a 200th or a 30th potency depending on the seriousness and the scope of the symptoms. The more fever the higher the potency; the more physical symptoms the lower the potency (Fig. 8.12).

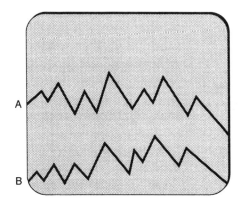

Fig. 8.12 Similarly, if B is the symptom picture of the remedy or the wave pattern created by this, and A is the disturbance pattern of the disease, B may not reach the activity level of A. Perhaps some parts – the high notes or peaks – may produce echoes that reach higher. These may touch and stimulate the octave above. Each musical instrument is different in tone and in the harmonies it produces, even though sounding the same notes as another.

THE EXPLANATION IN THIS SECTION IS A GREAT SIMPLIFICATION. THERE IS A CONSIDERABLE AMOUNT OF SKILL IN SELECTING A POTENCY, AND THIS IS BEST LEARNED THROUGH CLINICAL TRAINING.

ACTIVITY 3

1) Give a group of symptoms to which you would apply a 6th potency, a 30th potency, a 200th potency, a 1M potency and a 10M potency.
2) What symptoms of menstrual disorder might you expect to find were you to contemplate using the following potencies: 6th, 30th, 200th, 1M?
3) What potency would you use for the following symptoms? State your reasons.
   a. An ear discharging yellow pus
   b. A dog bite piercing the skin and drawing blood
   c. A girl hysterical with grief who cannot stop crying
   d. Itchy skin after eating very fresh tomatoes
   e. A septic toe, swollen and red
   f. A child who wakes screaming from a nightmare and cannot recognize anyone
   g. A cold wind causing toothache
   h. Fell and twisted an ankle
   i. Swollen left tonsil and smelly breath
   j. A blinding headache with severe nausea and red face
   k. Anger after being insulted by a shopkeeper; shouts and curses
   l. Warts on two fingers of the left hand
   m. Discharge from the right eye after being caught in a rainstorm
   n. Watery diarrhoea accompanied by severe cramps, tenesmus and fever
   o. Sneezes after falling in the river
   p. Heartburn only on lying down
   q. Trembling and loose bowel before exams
   r. Mood swings to violent temper before menses
   s. Severe burn causes blister covering the palm and searing pain; patient faints
   t. The hair falls out after childbirth, no other symptoms

The Collective Single Dose, the Ascending Collective Dose and the Split Dose

In the literature and in some practices it is common to find remedies used in these ways, and this is the best place to explain it.

Kent discovered that the use of the single dose could produce severe aggravation because there was too much reaction from the vital force. He gave another dose of medicine within a certain time period, which could then cut across the action of the remedy and slow it down. If the remedy produces a wave pattern of reaction, then a second remedy would cut across the outward-moving wave. The second remedy would be out of phase initially, and would deflect the vital force to bring it into phase, thus the main thrust of the remedy would be delayed.

The Collective Single Dose (CSD)

CSD is a total of three pills, given usually at 2 or 3-hourly intervals depending on how quickly the symptoms are moving. Sometimes it is given at 12 hours, or 6 hours. The faster the symptoms move, the closer together the doses.

The Split Dose (SD)

This is given immediately before sleep and is followed by another dose immediately on waking. Once again the phasing is put out, so that the reaction is slowed down. There is some mystical idea that, since only sleep comes between the doses, there is only one dose. It should be clear to you from what we have already discussed that this is not so. However, there are advantages in the procedure in some cases and it should not be disposed of so quickly.

The Ascending Collective Dose (ACD)

This is the name given to the process of giving three pills 2 or 3 hours apart, as in the CSD, but increasing the potency each time. Thus we might use a 6th potency, then the 30th then the 200th; or the 30th, then the 200th then the 1M potency. If we remember that the different potencies work on different octaves, and that action is needed on different energy levels to cure the patient, then this procedure can be likened to a starting handle, manually touching each level rather than waiting for the reaction of the vital force to do this in its own time. The procedure is again crude, but can be effective and useful in stimulating the level wanted, then quickly transferring the reaction to a higher, more free level, where less aggravation will occur.

ACTIVITY 4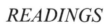

Study the diagram on page 192 of Vithoulkas' *The Science of Homoeopathy*. Write a few paragraphs relating what you now know of potency to your study of the importance of symptoms in the hierarchy. If you have one, a tutor will be very useful to help assess this work.

Explain the following in your own words. Check your answers with the text.

1) The lack of reaction to low potencies
2) Over-reaction to high potencies
3) The lack of reaction to higher potencies
4) The prolonged aggravation of lower potencies
5) The need to repeat lower potencies

READINGS

Hahnemann S *The organon*, paras 30–49, 58–62, 146–148, 154, 157–160, 245–257, 275–287

Kent J T *Lectures on homoeopathic philosophy*, Chs 36 & 37

FURTHER READING

Campbell A *1964 The two faces of homoeopathy*. Jain, New Delhi

LESSON NINE

Proving the Remedy

Headings: Introduction
What is a Proving?
Proving a Remedy
Exact Recording
Procedure
Quality of the Symptoms
A Complete Proving
Idiosyncrasy

Aim: By the end of this lesson you should be able to understand the legitimacy of the symptoms attached to a remedy symptom picture.

Objectives: To understand how a proving is conducted;
To understand how the remedy and the prover are prepared;
To be able to grade the quality of a symptom produced in a proving;
To be able to determine the suitability of provers.

Introduction

In order to practise homoeopathy, knowledge is required from three sources:

- The philosophy – the principles and practice of Homoeopathy;
- The Materia Medica of the remedy, the symptoms attached to the remedy;
- The patient – which knowledge is gained from case studies.

It is in the provings that knowledge of Materia Medica is gathered. Hahnemann in paras 19, 20 and 21 states that medicines by their very nature must have some power to alter our health, but this is not discovered by reasoning. The medicine must be observed in its action. The medicine must be administered to find its properties, as to how it can affect the health of an individual. There is no other way in which its character can be determined. As Hahnemann tells us in paras 118 and 119, each medicine is as unique as each plant is unique, or each element in the periodic table of elements is unique.

Homoeopathy is entirely rational and scientific in this acknowledgement. Each symptom ascribed to the symptom picture of a remedy has been observed in the proving of that remedy. The twelve volumes of Allen's *Encyclopedia of Materia Medica* contains lists of all symptoms produced by provers. It also contains lists of those symptoms produced by the remedy when taken accidentally. Whereas the poisoning symptoms are important and help us to understand the physiological action of the remedy, the proving is necessary to develop an idea of its dynamic action. In smaller doses, and in potentized form, the remedy acts on the vital force to unfold a pattern of disruption at many different levels of symptom, from the mental and emotional right down to the particular.

When you reach the finer stages of prescribing you will find Allen's volumes useful because he lists many cases there, and you can trace the disease pattern in its development. Also, since the very first provings, the exact words used by the prover (or the translation of this in some cases) have been retained, so we can get as close as possible to the original experience and thus accurately relate this to that of our patient. This explains why in many Materia Medica textbooks many phases keep recurring. This is not laziness on the part of the author, but is an attempt to preserve the original data. Unfortunately, our speech idiom today has changed, so the subtle feelings of the prover are often lost in archaic language. A tradition of clinical usage thus backs up the provings.

69

Kent frowned on the use of any homoeopathic remedy that had not been proved. In fact, both he and Hahnemann would have denied the label homoeopathic to such a practice. It is for this reason that many homoeopaths frown on the use of 'combination remedies': these mixtures have never been proved when so combined, so no one knows the exact effect of them.

What is a Proving?

This term is used to describe the process of observing the action of which a homoeopathic remedy is capable. The word comes from the German *prüfeng* meaning 'test'. The person taking the medicine is called the prover, and he or she must be a healthy individual. The medicine is given to the prover until he or she develops symptoms, then the administration of the medicine is stopped and the pattern of symptoms which develops is noted.

Homoeopathic remedies are never proved on animals or sick people. In the first instance an animal cannot speak or otherwise communicate; sick people are not used in provings quite simply because they already have a pattern of disturbance (they are ill, so how can one determine the effects due to the disturbance as opposed to those produced by the remedy?)

Proving a Remedy

The Stages of a Proving

1) The remedy is given to a healthy person until symptoms start to develop.
2) When symptoms develop the administration of the remedy is stopped.
3) The symptoms are noted as to precisely when and where they appear, and for 6 months to 1 year afterwards.
4) The recording of symptoms stops when no more symptoms appear and all those produced have disappeared again.
5) The data are collected and collated.
6) Further information is now needed from clinical experience of using the remedy.
7) The remedy's symptoms are entered in the repertories.

Criteria

Individuals will produce different results in the proving, and the type of symptoms and the speed with which they are produced will all depend on the potency used and the susceptibility of the individual. Some will be deeply affected by the remedy, others will not.

The proving will build up a picture of what type of person is affected by the remedy. In this a homoeopathic proving differs from a drug trial, because the homoeopath is looking for individuality whereas in the drug trial it is the statistical average of the drug's action which is sought.

The proving will show the dynamic action of the remedy as it affects the vital force, so individuality will be expressed in all groups of symptoms, from mental and emotional right through to particulars. Few homoeopathic provers will produce the strange, rare and peculiar symptoms, only those most susceptible to the drug. Yet these are the symptoms that most enable us to identify the remedy, because so few other remedies produce these symptoms.

Some symptoms will be heavily marked in all patients, and these will form the characteristic symptoms of the remedy and will be found in caricatures of the remedy.

Preparation

To ensure clarity in the results, we must prepare well to determine the purity of each stage of the proving. In this we are concerned with:

- The preparation of the remedy;
- The preparation of the Prover;
- The technique of exact recording and the assessment of the quality of the symptoms.

The last item will be dealt with in Lesson 11.

Preparation of the Remedy

Hahnemann the chemist was much concerned about the *purity* of the remedy to be tested, so he laid down the following rules:

- The plant must be fresh, even picked at a certain point in its lifecycle.
- Care must be taken that no foreign substance be introduced.
- The prover must take no other medicine that might lead to confusion – this includes almost all vegetables (see para 125) except potatoes, carrots, young peas and beans. For this reason all stimulating food such as tea, coffee, alcohol and spices were to be avoided, sometimes for a long time prior to proving. Later it was sufficient that the prover abstained for only 1 month prior to the proving.

Vithoulkas requires that remedies should be proven in different potencies in order to reveal all the hidden qualities. He attempts greater accuracy than Hahnemann and, by keeping apart the symptoms developed by each stage, he enables us to view more accurately the development of the disease process of each remedy. He also attempts to ensure a clearer mental and emotional picture by selecting only those provers sensitive to the remedy in its lower potencies to go on to participate in provings of the higher potencies. Of course, in terms of the allopathic testing of drugs we could say that Vithoulkas at this point ceases to be unbiased. In homoeopathic terms he is seeking those most susceptible to the remedy to bring out more individual symptoms.

The Preparation of the Prover

Selection of the Prover. The prover must also be in a state of 'purity', i.e. be capable of producing 'pure' symptoms. To accomplish this provers are selected according to the following criteria:

- They must be healthy.
- They must abstain from 'noxious habits' during and for a period before the proving.
- They must be intelligent and articulate in order to recognize and clearly record symptoms.

Vithoulkas also requires that the whole sample should be balanced as regards sex and age, and he undertakes the proving at 1500 feet above sea level to eliminate extremes of atmospheric pressure.

Before the Proving Kent has each prover examine him or herself for 1 week prior to the proving, and take careful notes of their usual habits. This is an excellent idea, as many are so out of touch with the body's many symptoms or individual character that some peculiarities go unnoticed until attention is focused on them. It would give a false reading if these were discovered during a proving.

Vithoulkas sends provers to 1500 feet, where sea level and high altitude are balanced (see Vithoulkas, *The Science of Homoeopathy*, page 150). The prover is stabilized for 15 days, environmental factors are neutralized, and again the prover writes down the symptoms, as with Kent's procedure, but this time Vithoulkas assesses provers ruthlessly. He omits anyone:

- Who wrote down a lot of mental and emotional symptoms;
- Who omitted to recall symptoms;
- Who exhibited superficiality in reporting symptoms;
- Who suffered from hypersensitivity diseases.

In doing this he takes out any prover who is easily influenced, giving them placebos and using them as part of the control group. The old homoeopaths would argue that he might miss an area of the remedy's activity, and indeed with certain remedies (the most sensitive) he might have difficulty obtaining a good proving simply because he has taken out those who are most susceptible to that type of remedy! However, Vithoulkas must be complimented that his procedure is very clear and lends itself to accuracy and precision in gathering data.

During the Proving. A supervisor will check up on the prover to ascertain that he or she is following the procedure and is accurately recording all symptoms. The supervisor will also check on the health of the prover during the proving.

Vithoulkas insists on double-blind trials, in which neither the prover nor the supervisor is aware which remedy is being proved, or indeed which prover has been given the remedy rather than a placebo.

A Biased Sample

A modern scientific researcher might well find Hahnemann's procedure biased. Although his instruction to avoid stressful situations and any over-exertion might be seen as valid, his request for only intelligent persons who could describe sensations accurately might cause a few raised eyebrows. His request for self-observation and introspection of such a degree would no doubt raise cries of interference in data production. One who was looking for symptoms so intensely would no doubt find them, it could be argued, whether or not they were present. The latter could be overcome by using double-blind techniques and even by the isolation of provers, so that they could not communicate and contaminate each other's data.

Although these allegations are certainly justifiable, I usually silence such by giving them a remedy and a sealed envelope containing its name. Then after they have produced enough symptoms, instruct them to open the envelope and refer to the relevant page of a Materia Medica textbook published over a century ago. As it is an infallible procedure, they will find their symptoms described in detail by an earlier prover. Whether scientific or not by today's standards, the proving procedure has given valuable facts on which homoeopathy's record of cure has rested for almost 2 centuries.

It should be noted, though, that homoeopathy fulfils the ultimate scientific criterion in that the experiment is repeatable. One serious drawback in conducting provings today is that individuals are more chronically ill than in Hahnemann's day, so it may be difficult to find individuals who are healthy enough.

Vithoulkas has added a great deal of accuracy to the proving procedure, putting it into a more logical framework and bringing it into line with the requirements of today's drug trials. The last word, however, must go to Hahnemann, who in para 133 requests *ingenuity* of the prover. When the symptom arrives the prover is expected to experiment with all sorts of positions and conditions, to determine as much as possible the modalities that affect the symptom, i.e. what makes it worse and what makes it better.

Exact Recording

The prover recording the symptoms must use clarity, simplicity and precision. Hahnemann tells us to record the simple language and the exact words of the prover. As previously mentioned, this is invaluable to preserve a record as close as possible to the original in meaning and nuance. The prover writes down the symptoms every day for Hahnemann, whereas Vithoulkas requires them written down three times each day, in case the prover forgets.

Accuracy is aided by the use of a schema such as that used by Clark in his Materia Medica dictionary. Thus at each recording the prover will go over each item in the schema: are there any symptoms in the head, eyes, ears, throat, chest, skin, etc? Symptoms at all levels and in all parts of the body and psyche must be recorded, and this schema helps the prover realize the scope of the remedy's possible action and, of course, aids lapses of memory.

A diagram of the body is useful to help the location of symptoms. The prover is not expected to have an exact knowledge of anatomy and physiology, and here the supervisor comes in to help.

Each symptom should be completed as far as possible according to time, location, sensation and modality, in order that the symptoms produced will be of maximum use to the homoeopath. Once again the supervisor may aid by providing an understanding of homoeopathic needs.

Procedure

The aim of the proving is to produce symptoms. Once the prover has been prepared, the remedy is administered. There are different ways to do this. Hahnemann gives a 30th potency each day in the form of four to six small globules on an empty stomach. Another common practice is to administer just one pill or tablet of a high-potency remedy. With lower potencies the remedy may be ingested every 15 minutes, or every hour, until change occurs.

Once reaction of any kind sets in the remedy is ceased, and under no circumstance whatever does the prover restart after stopping.

Though the medicine is no longer being taken, its action continues as the vital force accommodates the disturbance, so the prover goes on recording symptoms for 6 months or even a year (see Appendix for a copy of the Society of Homoeopaths Proving Instructions to Supervisors and Provers).

Quality of the Symptoms

Susceptibility

By its very nature the medicine will affect the health of an individual and so will eventually disturb the vital force of almost anyone producing symptoms, according to the nature of the remedy. The actual symptoms may vary slightly according to the weakness that the vital force disturbed, e.g. if we take Belladonna it will produce heat and fever, dryness and redness, as part of its general characteristics in the proving, but one individual with weakness in the eyes will produce the dilated pupils of Belladonna more readily than another, who may produce congestive headache or swollen tonsils more readily. The prover will react to the remedy according to his or her weaknesses (constitutional predisposition) and susceptibility. If the prover is very susceptible to the remedy (resonates strongly with it), only one dose may be necessary to produce the symptoms (para 129). You will also find that *someone who is very susceptible to the remedy will produce symptoms very quickly.*

In some provers the symptoms produced will continue into a deeper level, but may only do so if the disturbance is continued by repeated doses of the remedy. The remedy may also affect more deeply if the vitality is lowered. Thus, unlike patients, healthy provers often need more than one dose before the remedy takes hold.

The Quality of the Reaction

The best proving is when reaction comes after the first dose. When this happens there is an order to the symptoms that shows a developmental stage of the remedy (see para 130, and Vithoulkas's *Science of Homoeopathy* page 145, action and reaction). This is important, as it enables us to recognize the remedy in the patient before it necessarily reaches a crisis situation. Such a proving may also show two actions of the medicine: the primary action of the disturbance (which is often invisible in the prodromal stages of the disease), and the second reaction of the vital force to correct the balance by throwing out symptoms according to its resonance with the remedy.

In order to ensure the possibility of the first reaction, Kent recommends waiting until the duration of action of the remedy is completed, if this is known. Hence in his proving he may use a single dose of high potency. Facts become lost when one wave is started after another and time for reaction is not allowed. The disturbance has increased greatly and subtle symptoms are lost. If the duration of action of the remedy is not known, then there is difficulty.

When the action period has elapsed without a reaction, Kent advises taking the 30th potency every 2 hours until a reaction occurs. This, he says, intensifies the effect and shortens the prodromal period. This gap can be shortened or lengthened to speed up or slow down the build-up of disturbance, but once again it is important not to stop taking the remedy and then restart.

Kent also suggests that it is important to take enough of a drug to disturb the vital force but not to suspend it. Sometimes in treatment we can recognize that continued treatment may produce no symptoms because each dose, or in some cases each change of remedy, interferes with the first before the reaction of the vital force appears. In some cases, in fact, it appears as if the patient gets worse all the time, as the new remedies are allowed to produce primary reactions to the disturbance but not the second action of correction. How can this be applied to the proving situation? It is necessary to choose a strong enough potency to create reaction, hence Hahnemann's use of the 30th potency. It is also necessary to allow sufficient time between each dose, hence Hahnemann's allowance of 24 hours, only decreasing this time gap if reaction was slow.

A Complete Proving

Vithoulkas divided the proving into three sections.

- After first observing the patient's natural symptoms for 1 month or 15 days, he gave a hypertoxic dose three times daily for 1 month, or until symptoms appeared. Twenty-five percent are given placebo. He expected different reactions to the remedy depending on the provers' susceptibility: those susceptible will quickly produce symptoms and these will probably be sufficiently numerous to distinguish this group from others. This group of susceptibles is used in proving the higher potencies because they are more sensitive to the remedy.
- After a long gap the remedy is taken by the group of susceptibles in the 30th potency daily for 2 weeks, or until symptoms appear. Again, twenty-five percent are given placebo. Once again the most susceptible will react quickly and intensely. This new group of susceptibles will do a further proving 1 year later, using the 10M or 50M potency.
- Only one pill is given and the patient is observed for 3 months until symptoms cease. Again, twenty-five percent are given placebo.

Hahnemann and Kent were content that the proving was complete when no new symptoms could be elicited from the provers (para 135). To Vithoulkas the proving was complete only when

- Three levels of potency were proved (i.e. the toxic, hypotoxic and high potency levels);
- Three levels of symptoms were produced (i.e. S, R & P, general, and mental and emotional);
- Clinical evidence proved that the remedy could cure the symptoms produced.

In the modern scientific world, Vithoulkas' criteria are more acceptable because they exhaust all possibilities that the remedy could produce, and also because of greater precision and accuracy.

Of course, we do not poison the patient. Many homoeopathic remedies are very violent poisons in their crude dose, and there are many examples of such poisonings. They produce primarily physical changes in health, i.e. changes in physiology. Allen's encyclopedia includes this information, gathered from accidental poisonings, as well as the provings. The poisonings may be useful to show how the remedy may be applied to advanced stages of pathology. It could be said that such poisonings represent the final stages of the disease process of the remedy. Of course, the homoeopath does not need to wait to treat the patient until pathological changes occur. Poisonings usually involve massive doses that swamp the life processes within the body. The potentized dose is much more diluted, and so affects the organism without causing death or physiological change.

ACTIVITY 1 Write a paragraph in answer to the questions below, showing you understand the principles involved. A tutor will help you assess this, or you may discuss the theories with colleagues.

1) 'Not all symptoms are produced equally by all provers'. Discuss.
2) One individual will not produce all the symptoms of the remedy at any one time. Discuss. (Para 134 may help)
3) During a proving all sick people are cured. Discuss. (Para 117 may help)

4) Why does the prover's health always improve after the remedy? (Para 141, Kent's *Lectures in Homoeopathic Philosophy*, page 208 and Vithoulkas *The Science of Homoeopathy*, page 146 may help)

5) Why do the prover's chronic symptoms disappear after undertaking a proving, perhaps to reappear later. (See Kent, page 208)

6) If there is no sensitivity, how can we create sensitivity? (See Vithoulkas, pages 146 and 154)

7) Why is a break in the proving dangerous? (See Kent, Chapter 28)

ACTIVITY 2 Write full instructions for a prover to follow during a proving. Compare this with the directions given by Jeremy Sheer. (See appendix II)

ACTIVITY 3 Discuss the homoeopathic proving as a scientific procedure.
This is a good exercise to discuss in a group.
The readings may help.

Idiosyncrasy

This word crops up frequently in homoeopathic literature; it refers to the patient's individual characteristics. One almost says susceptibilities, and then asks, what is the difference?

On the surface there is no difference between susceptibility, predisposition and idiosyncrasy: the way in which the patient is resonant is predisposition; the degree to which he or she is resonant is susceptibility; idiosyncrasy is that to which the patient is sensitive, i.e. resonates. Today we might call such sensitivity allergies. Kent tells us some are inherited and some acquired. We may only truly get rid of those inherited if the underlying miasm or predisposition is treated. To be specific, Kent says that sensitivities are due to psora and need antipsoric treatment.

In the proving, the peculiar idiosyncrasies of the remedy are exposed and it is this individual characteristic that we look for in patients.

READINGS

Hahnemann S *The organon*, paras 105–145, 118–146
Kent J T *Lectures on homoeopathic philosophy*, Chs 28, 29, 30, 31
Vithoulkas G *The science of homoeopathy*, Chs 10, 18 and Appendix A

Taking the Case

Headings: Introduction
The Aim of Case-Taking
The Interview Technique
Recording the Case
Causation

Aims: At the end of this lesson the student will have a basic theory of case-taking, i.e. the interview technique and the recording skills. A little practice is then needed.

Objectives: To understand the aim of case-taking;
To know the type of question that will not bias the symptoms obtained;
To develop a method of recording data.

Introduction

Taking the case is eliciting symptoms from the patient. It is finding out:

- What is the matter (para 3);
- What is to be cured in disease (para 7);
- The disturbance of the vital force, the total symptom picture (para 17);
- The totality of the disease.

It is the interview with the patient.
The information needed by the homoeopath falls into three categories:

- Knowledge of homoeopathic philosophy and principles of practice;
- Knowledge of homoeopathic Materia Medica;
- Knowledge of the patient.

Taking the case is the third of these categories.
Obtaining the symptoms is the homoeopathic process of examination of the patient. The first interview usually takes at least 1 hour, and may even take 2 or 3 unless the case is acute, in which case speed may be important. It is a labour-intensive process of obtaining objective and subjective symptoms, but such a degree of accuracy and detail is required that interview techniques and skills have been developed. In this lesson we will look at these techniques and examine the criteria used to judge the quality of the information.

The Aim of Case-Taking

The aim of case taking is to achieve good reliable prescribing symptoms. These enable us to:

- Select a remedy;
- Make a good choice of potency;
- Assess the need for any other appropriate treatment.

To achieve this end we need:

- Accuracy
- Precision
- Objectivity

Accuracy

Do we understand what the patient is saying? This is not as obvious as it may seem. For example, the patient may say she is afraid of crowds. There are many ways in which this can be interpreted – claustrophobia, dislike of being touched, desire to escape, or to hide herself, oversensitivity of feelings.

When we take down the patient's symptoms we always do so in his or her own words, because it enables us to go back and reinterpret the data if necessary.

Precision

In exactly which part of the head is the pain?
In exactly which direction is the pain shooting?

In the abdominal section of the Repertory, Kent uses three words for locations which are very close to each other: ilium, inguinal and iliosacral. The practitioner should know which is which. The patient is not expected to know anatomical names and locations, so must always be asked to point to the place. Assumption gives rise to false information.

Objectivity

We need to remain uncoloured by our own prejudices, yet we seek that which is strange, rare and peculiar. In fact, Kent tells us we have no case if there are no peculiars, but how do we judge what is normal? What is normal to us or what is normal to the culture in which we live may be odd to some patients. Deviation from the norm is already a relative concept.

In our work we are looking for the whole of the patient, including his or her subjectivity, but subjectivity is not just the patient saying 'I feel'; it is also listening to attitude and perspective, which requires special skills of the practitioner and a vast knowledge of self!

Hahnemann speaks of case-taking in para 83, in which he says

'it . . . demands nothing but freedom from prejudice and sound senses, attention in observing and fidelity in tracing the picture of the disease'.

On page 180, Vithoulkas says

'. . . the primary goal is to accurately and precisely describe all the important factors in the case, while eliminating irrelevant information'. He also adds that '. . . the record should communicate the relative intensity of emphasis of particular symptoms'.

Kent, on page 198, says

'The purpose of all this is that you will go away and examine the patient with an unprejudiced mind, that you will consider only the case before you, that you will have nothing in mind that will distract your attention, that you may not think of things that preceded it and find out from among them a remedy while examining the patient. If you are biased in your judgement and examine the patient towards a certain remedy, in many instances this will prove to be fatal. Have no remedy in mind until you have everything that you can get on paper. Have it all written down carefully and then if, upon examining it in relation to remedies, you are unable to distinguish between three or four, you can go back and re-examine the patient with references to those three or four remedies'.

THE OBJECT OF CASE-TAKING IS TO GAIN FROM THE PATIENT A VIEW OF THE OVERALL PATTERN OF HOW THE VITAL FORCE IS EXPRESSED IN THIS INDIVIDUAL. THIS COVERS MENTAL, EMOTIONAL AND PHYSICAL SPHERES AND HOW ALL THESE FIT TOGETHER TO MAKE A PATTERN, INCLUDING OVER TIME, WHICH WE KNOW AS THE TOTAL SYMPTOM PICTURE.

You must also keep in mind what Kent said, (page 229), that pages and pages of symptoms do not necessarily make a case – it is prescribing symptoms we are looking for.

Case-taking boils down to two factors:

1) Seeking that which is most individual in the patient, (para 84);
2) Seeking that point of change where the vital force was disturbed or altered.

The Interview Technique

Hahnemann mentions certain conditions that should surround the process of case taking; Kent puts this into even more detail, likening the practitioner's skills to those of a lawyer questioning a witness in court. Vithoulkas uses modern psychotherapy to refine the art yet further. We will look at the information that must be acquired, and the means by which this may be done.

The Information

This falls into four categories, which naturally follow each other during the case-taking procedure:

1) Listening to the patient's presenting symptoms;
2) Clarifying and completing each symptom in homoeopathic parlance;
3) Interviewing the patient to find the total symptom picture;
4) The observations of the homoeopath and of relatives or others close to the patient.

The Presenting Symptoms

From Hahnemann, the first rule is for the practitioner to keep silent, allowing the patient to express symptoms in his or her own language. Left without interruption, it is also likely that the patient will order the complaints according to how important they are in his or her experience, i.e. depending on intensity, how much they affect everyday life and so on. There is also a great deal of information to be obtained from how the patient describes symptoms, so the homoeopath remains silent so as not to lose this information.

PRACTICE POINT

There are, however, difficulties the practitioner should be aware of:

1) *Conditioned Language*
   In this day and age the patient's attitude to his or her symptoms has been conditioned by allopathic medicine.
   The patient has been taught a language with which to express symptoms.
   The patient has been given an idea that certain symptoms are important while others are not – unfortunately the 'unimportant' are often those that are important to homoeopaths, i.e. subjective sensations.
   The patient has been taught by allopathy that symptoms are unnatural and should be got rid of, so often the patient has taken a drug, or vitamins or other therapies which cause symptoms to disappear or be distorted, or it may be the patient has no idea of modalities, of how the body feels, because he simply takes an asprin.

2) *Language Masking Symptoms*
   Also in this modern era, psychotherapy as a folk culture has encouraged the patient to express feelings in specific ways, or to rationalize these rather than feel them – Vithoulkas gives good examples of this. Other examples might be: 'yes, I'm feeling awful but you should see what I'm putting up with at work, or at home, or . . .' 'I understand X is going through a difficult time so I don't get angry, or I do something else with my anger, or worries, or fears'. The patient's feelings are modified, sublimated in some of these examples, suppressed or explained away in a manner similar to drugging or vitamin therapy.

3) *Emotional Exaggeration*
   Kent was only worried about the exaggeration of symptoms in the hypochondriac, or symptoms unexpressed through shyness, or the trend of false modesty in those days. We still see all of these today, and more.

Completing the Patient Symptoms

If the patient does not remember new material when prompted with the question, 'anything else?', then the practitioner's next job is to go over all the material presented by the patient and fill out each symptom according to:

- Time
- Location
- Sensation
- Modality
- Intensity

(See Lesson 4).

When recording the data, as the patient tells it, each symptom is put on a fresh line and enough space is left to go back and fill in the details when the patient has finished speaking (*Organon*, paras 86 and 87).

Presenting symptoms are those about which the patient is worried, and the patient must be satisfied at the end of the interview that these have been dealt with satisfactorily.

The Total Symptom Picture

Since we are looking for the total symptom picture, we must concern ourselves with *how the patient copes with life*, how he or she interacts with the environment, the quality of life, the mental stages, the functions of the body – the *constitutional picture* (see paras 88 and 89).

Each case is unique, and areas to be further explored usually arise out of the conversation quite naturally. However, when faced with a totally blank face, because the patient does not know what is expected of him or her, or even after an explanation, a technique, or at least an opener, is required from the homoeopath. The three techniques below also indicate the scope of the material required in case-taking.

Using a straightforward schema. A schema, as in Kent's Repertory or Clarke's Materia Medica, enables one to cover all parts of the organism, i.e. mind, vertigo, head, eyes, vision, ears etc. This looks at the body in terms of space, and may involve such questions as 'What is your history of eye problems?' or 'When did you last have digestive problems and what were these?' This may be useful in opening up the allopathically trained patient.

Looking at the body as a functioning organism. Some bodily processes are more amenable to change than others. These fall under two headings, the excretory processes and assimilation processes.

Excretory processes	Assimilation processes
Defecation	Digestion
Urination	Learning
Sweat	Understanding
Respiration	Sleep
	Respiration

In these processes the greatest daily change takes place. The excretory processes are necessary for health, and particularly relevant in disease, so they are often brought in to do 'overtime'.

The bodily processes can also be evaluated according to their contribution to the whole. Disturbance in some parts is more serious than in others, so this technique helps us to apply the Law of Cure inversely to show the depth of disturbance. For example, the preservation of the species is more fundamental than the preservation of the individual, so disturbance in the reproduction system affecting desire, menstruation, etc. shows a more serious problem than disturbance in the ears, eyes, throat, etc.

Similarly, certain functions, e.g. sleep and appetite, are under less voluntary control because they are more primitive or vital, and thus again show deeper, more fundamental problems if disturbed. Many of these functions fall into the category of general symptoms. Other functions under more conscious control and therefore subject to more individual difference, may be less vital.

The effect of external factors and functions such as the weather, astronomy, the seasons, the environment and overall energy, could also be considered as representing the general level of symptom and therefore the body as a whole.

PRACTICE POINT   Overall energy, the force, vitality, or how the patient feels, is a sound criterion of progress during treatment, and is an element in selecting potency.

Historical Perspective. This involves building up the historical picture of the changes in the vital force; thus the questioning may start and work its way back through time, or it may mean concentrating on the picture of change produced at a particular time, checking to see how it has changed.

Of course these methods are usually intermingled, and the particular relevance of any one depends on the actual case treated. The value of delineating such procedures here is simply to give the beginner some idea of possibilities.

The Observations

The practitioner's observations are added last (para 90). The trained person knows what to look for. The patient's environment is full of clues to lifestyle and to what is important to this individual. The clothes and mannerisms tell of culture that may need to be accounted for when evaluating the symptoms; for example, very loose clothing may not point to Lachesis as the remedy if these are in fashion, or black clothing may not point to Platina as the remedy if the patient is an Arab lady who traditionally dresses in black.

The posture may be important in an acute or chronic case, perhaps giving clues as to the modalities. An open window, or a water jug half empty beside the bed, may give modalities that the distraught patient is unaware of or cannot concentrate on.

In the acute case, the study of the patient's immediate environment is most valuable.

In the chronic case the patient's tension may be evident in his body, even though he says adamantly that he is easygoing and has no worries. Anything the patient says adamantly may be a cover-up! A little hesitation, a gentle sigh can point out areas of sensitivity the patient may not volunteer, or may not be able to express.

In work with children, the practitioner must observe because there is a lot a child cannot say.

In this section we should also include information from relatives or the nurse attending the patient. Care must be taken, though, not to admit hearsay as evidence and to look for fact, judging opinion by its relevance to the experience of the observer.

The Questions

Once the patient has finished speaking, it is the homoeopath's turn, and both Kent and Vithoulkas are very clear that we should conduct ourselves in such a way as not to influence the patient, and that all questions should be directed in an open manner. In this way we follow where the patient leads, and we allow the patient always to express what is foremost in his or her mind.

Here are the rules:

- *No leading questions:* some people are easily influenced, are confused, or are too ready to please.
- *No questions with yes/no answers:* this is too black and white and tells us too little; the patient does not need to think or explore sensations or feelings.
- *No direct questions:* for the same reason as above, although these are admissible at the later stage when the case is nearly full but the remedy still needs to be differentiated within a small group of remedies.
- *Questions giving a choice of answer:* why? How do we know the relevance to the patient? How many options have we left out, one of which might be more important.

81

- *Do not hurry the patient:* tune into his or her rhythm and experience it, because this is part of your prescription. It is also essential for the patient's clarity not to rush, nor to confuse so that something is left out. There is nothing more frustrating than the patient telephoning to tell you another symptom that changes your prescription, especially when you have already given a remedy! Suspect a poorly taken case.
- *Allow the patient to finish one sentence before starting another:* the above comments apply here.
- *Do not question along the lines of a remedy:* as well as influencing the patient you will colour all the facts and distort your own judgement.

Recording the Case

The purpose here is obviously preservation of the data, but we must also retain some sense of the attitude and atmosphere of the patient. We need to preserve information about the symptoms as expressed by the patient. We need a note of presenting symptoms and prescribing symptoms, and what treatment was given and the patient's response to treatment.

Information must be ordered in such a way that it is easily retrievable. You must also be able to write it down easily while the patient is talking. A number of devices make this simpler.

- Hahnemann advises starting each symptom on a fresh line and leaving space to go back and fill in the details when time permits. This enables information to be grouped together, and must be a fundamental part of any system.
- Vithoulkas uses the method of underlining so the information stands out, if important or stressed.
- Joseph Revers, an Israeli homoeopath, advises that the page should be organized into four or five columns, according to how each symptom relates to Kent's repertory.

Vithoulkas' Underlining Method

Vithoulkas adds a great deal to the art of case-taking with his idea of underlining, which enables us to obtain a more three-dimensional approach or energy level. Some remedies may have the same symptoms but differ in their intensity. His idea is to look at each symptom in terms of clarity, intensity (of symptom) and spontaneity (was it volunteered by the patient?). A symptom which has all three of these factors is given three underlines, whereas a symptom that has none is not underlined. One underline may denote the symptom is clear but not intense, and not volunteered by the patient but obtained under questioning. Two underlines may be clear and spontaneously volunteered, but not intense. The system is very useful because symptoms stand out from the page and enable the homoeopath to concentrate on the most significant items. It also encourages the homoeopath in the habit of continually assessing the quality of the information. One disadvantage might be that the patient sees the homoeopath underlining, and that this may influence him or her, so distorting information and undoing the work of all that silence.

Joseph Rever's Column Method

Main section of repertory	Rubric	Modality	Remarks or space for patient's own words	Review of symptoms
Stomach	Appetite	Lacking at night	As if just eaten	Date 2/2/92 xxx three days after remedy
Stomach	Desires	Salt	This has been present since she had flu last year	2/2/92 disappeared after remedy
		Pork		

As the information is retrieved from the patient it is entered into one of the five columns. First, the homoeopath asks 'under which section of the Repertory will I find this symptom?' This section is then entered into the first column. 'How is the symptom to be looked up in the Repertory?' What rubric is to be used? This goes into the second column. 'What else do I know about the symptom?' Time, location, sensation and modality are entered one under the other in the third column. Any particularly interesting phrases or words used by the patient are entered in the fourth column, and the fifth is unused in the initial consultation. In subsequent consultations, when the homoeopath goes over all the symptoms, any change will be entered in the fifth column.

This seems a very easy process, producing clear information, especially if we also underline the symptoms as in the Vithoulkas method above. The system is very useful for a beginner, as you have to think–'What is the patient saying, what does that mean, do I need to know more of that symptom before it is useful?' Following this method you will not end up with pages and pages of vague useless information. Things come to mind during the interview when there is still the time to ask the patient, or it is possible to clarify ambiguous information because the case takes shape during the interview.

Red Asterisk

I often add red asterisks to mark symptoms I have used as prescribing symptoms to select the remedy. These are not usually added at the time of case-taking, but afterwards during the case analysis. They are useful in recalling the way I saw things at the time, especially when I go back to the case after a time lapse.

Other Information

Other information that needs to be recorded is of course, name, address, telephone number, date of birth, occupation, date of visit, and all this belongs at the beginning of the case notes in order to identify the patient. Occupation may tell us the type of environment or stress the patient is exposed to. The home situation, spouse and number of children can also be useful. The remedies given and the treatment recommended is recorded at the end of each visit. It may be useful to summarize this on a separate record card for easy access during telephone conversations or acute crisis.

ACTIVITY 1
The only way to absorb this material is to apply it, so practise taking some cases.
Experiment with different ways of asking questions.
Use different ways of recording the information.
Always make sure that each symptom is 'completed'.
TAKE AT LEAST TWO CASES.

Causation

In speaking of causation we are recognizing the point of change, or those factors such as exciting or maintaining causes that cause change.

Causation is often found as a section at the end of some Materia Medicas, e.g. Clarke's and Boenninghausen's. In Kent's Repertory, causation is to be found in the General section as modalities.

When we look over a case it might become obvious that there was *one point after which the symptom picture appeared*. An event preceding this point may become obvious as 'a cause', something that was able to affect the health of a patient, i.e. able to disturb the vital force. This is the exciting cause. Thus a blow with a blunt instrument may produce a deterioration in health. The vital force may quickly resolve the situation so that the only remedy required is first-aid, or it may be that the vital force is knocked off centre so a new point of balance is attempted. If this happens, the patient will develop a new set of symptoms after the accident and this may obscure the cause.

After a situation of grief a patient may develop anxiety attacks, arthritis, multiple sclerosis or cancer, etc. This new symptom picture may be treated with the same remedy as the grief, or it may be treated with a different remedy because the symptom picture is different. In this last case the problem may well improve, but often it will never fully resolve until the real problem, the suppressed grief, is treated. In some cases this is easy because the remedy for the exciting cause and the new symptom picture are the same.

Arnica produces symptoms similar to a blunt instrument injury, namely bruising or aching all over. The remedy at the time of injury may have been Arnica, but if the vital force cannot overcome the trauma it will lock it safely away, and as it does so it will change octaves so that what becomes too dangerous to display in the acute level will be expressed at a deeper level in the more chronic but less threatening manner. The new picture may or may not be similar to Arnica's symptom picture. The original Arnica picture may merge with the constitutional picture to produce a more complex disease – the merging of two miasms – or might simply enhance the constitutional picture. If the symptom picture joins with another, the result may resemble neither Arnica nor the constitutional remedy. There may be a third picture, but the remedy that appears to be indicated by the camouflaged picture may not be able to cure if it cannot resonate with the Arnica level, i.e. the exciting cause or point of change. *When we treat homoeopathically it is not the symptoms that are treated, but what disturbed the vital force.* In cure, the disturbance of the vital force is resolved. Thus we must prescribe for the causation. In the best-fit remedy this will also include the total symptom picture or reaction to the point of change.

READINGS

Kent J T *Lectures on homoeopathic philosophy*, Chs 22, 23, 24, 25, 26 & 27
Vithoulkas G *The science of homoeopathy*, Ch. 12

ADDITIONAL READING

Nash E B *How to take a case.* Jain, New Delhi
Schmidt P *1976 The act of interrogation.* Homoeopathic Medical Pub, Bombay
Schmidt P *1976 The act of case taking.* Homoeopathic Medical Pub, Bombay

LESSON ELEVEN

The Repertory

Headings: Role of the Repertory
Different Repertories
The Organization of the Repertory

Aim: Before concentrating on Kent's Repertory, this chapter will provide you with an overview.

Objectives: To recognize the styles of Repertory;
To recognize how symptoms are ordered in Kent's Repertory;
To be able to find a symptom in a Repertory.

Role of the Repertory

The Repertory is one of the most valuable tools the homoeopath possesses. It is a dictionary of symptoms and after each symptom are listed the remedies known to cause that symptom in the proving. Since there are over 2000 homoeopathic remedies, the Repertory helps us to select the remedy more accurately.

Different Repertories

There are numerous Repertories. Some are tagged on to volumes of Materia Medica, and others are complex works by themselves. Some Repertories in common use are:

Barthel H 1987 The synthetic repertory. Jain, New Delhi

Boericke W 1987 Homoeopathic materia medica with repertory. Homoeopathic Book Service, Sittingbourne

Clarke C J 1988 A clinical repertory to the dictionary of materia medica. Jain, New Delhi

Hering C 1988 Analytical repertory of mind symptoms. Jain, New Delhi

Kent J T 1986 Repertory of homoeopathic materia medica. Jain, New Delhi

Phatak S R 1963 A concise repertory of homoeopathic remedies. Devaki Enterprises, Bombay

Roberts H A, Wilson A 1985 Von Boenninghausen's repertory of materia medica. Jain, New Delhi

The Organization of the Repertory

The most commonly used are Phatak's and Kent's, and these illustrate two different styles of arranging the symptoms.

Phatak's Repertory

This is more like a dictionary, with each symptom arranged alphabetically. It is based on Kent's Repertory but is much smaller, and contains only the most common remedies in each rubric.

The remedies are entered under the rubrics in Kent's three grades of type, namely **bold**, *italic* and ordinary. Its great value is that Phatak culls from his clinical experience, listing useful 'everyday' symptoms such as high blood pressure. To find this in Kent you must look up all the component symptoms, such as:

- Bursting headache
- Palpitations

- Epistaxis
- Oedema

Kent never allows you to think of anything but individuality. Working in India long after Kent, Phatak adds many useful minor remedies to his lists. Some of these have long been in use in Indian pharmacopoeias and have clinical value, but are sometimes poorly proved, e.g. Ceanthus.

Kent's Repertory

Kent's Repertory is almost 100 years old. It has been updated several times by notable homoeopaths, including Boericke, the latest being additions by Vithoulkas based on his clinical experience of 20 000 cases. There are several editions of Kent's Repertory, a final general edition containing all additions except Vithoulkas'.

The basis of Kent's Repertory is the homoeopathic provings. The symptoms that are listed are those which appear in the provings, and grades are attached to each remedy appearing under a symptom, depending on how important that particular symptom was in the proving.

- **Heavy black type.** If a symptom is printed in heavy black type, almost all provers will produce this symptom in the provings. Thus it is also strongly marked in the symptom picture of the patient who requires this remedy.
- *Italic type.* Italics indicate that a large proportion of provers produce this symptom, and the remedy has consistently shown that it is capable of curing that symptom.
- Ordinary type. This indicates that only a minority of provers produced this symptom in the proving, and the remedy's ability to cure the symptom is as yet by no means validated in clinical experience.

Clinical experience, it should be noted, can be used to update the entry of a remedy under any symptom. Almost all Repertories use the grades of type adopted by Kent. Boenninghausen is the exception to this. He uses five categories variously represented by asterisks and capitals in different editions. Boenninghausen predates Kent, and his Repertory was the first to attempt to grade the remedies.

Schematic Order

In his Repertory Kent follows Boenninghausen's style of dividing symptoms into a schema representing different parts of the body. In Kent, all the mental and emotional symptoms are found in the first part of the Repertory under Mind. The generalities are found at the end of the Repertory, and these contain many modalities and exciting causes. In between these two parts, Kent starts at the top of the body and works through the parts. Vertigo is a product of dysfunctioning consciousness and is found in a separate section after Mind.

In principle Kent often followed the section of a 'part' with its product, e.g.

- Rectum – Stool
- Bladder – Urine
- Chest – Expectoration

Sometimes, as in Menses, Vomit and Catarrh, the product is found under the appropriate part. There is no justification for this difference.

The parts start with the Head, Eyes, Ears, Throat, Stomach, Abdomen, Genitalia, back up to the Larynx, Chest, and then Back Extremities, etc.

ACTIVITY 1   List Kent's schema in order. Note how he comes down the front of the body into the stomach, back up and down into the chest, back up and down the back.
Note which products of metabolism have their own sections.
Why do you think sleep, skin and perspiration are at the end before Generalities?
When would you use the chill and fever section?

Alphabetical Order of Rubrics

Once we have found the main section in Kent's Repertory, each rubric is then listed alphabetically, e.g. Mind,   Abandoned,
                                                                                    Abrupt,
                                                                                    Absent-minded . . .

To find things easily in the Repertory you can ask two questions: 'Where is this symptom located?' will give you the section of the Repertory, and 'What is happening in the part?' will help you to label the rubric.

TLSM

After each rubric comes its specifics, which Kent has ordered: first time, then location, sensation and modalities. This order never varies and is to be found throughout the Repertory.

If we wish to find a pain in the arm, we will look up Extremities as the section and Pain as the rubric. Next, under the sensation Pain come the modalities, i.e. what aggravates or ameliorates the pain. Then we have a problem! Arm is a further sublocation under Extremities, and it follows the modalities of pain. This order can be very confusing for the uninitiated, but look at the order:

- Location Extremities
- Sensation Pain
- Modality then Location again.

The symptoms are ordered wheel within wheel, going into more precise location and greater detail. This is the map, and if you remember it you will not get lost (Fig. 11.1).

Note that sensations and modalities are arranged alphabetically, but once again location starts at the top and works down, so upper limbs come before lower limbs. Upper limbs start at the shoulder, working down through the upper arm, elbow, arm, wrist, hand, palm, thumb and fingers, whilst the lower limbs start at the hip and work down through the nates (buttocks), thigh, knee, leg, foot, heel, sole and toes. Nails appear on the fingers and toes, as expected. Tendons, tibia, calf and relevant muscles also appear where expected.

Note that not all symptoms are complete symptoms. Is there a location for constipation? What is the sensation of nausea? Sometimes part of TLSM is left out. In the example given, pain in the arm, each stage of the wheel may not be repeated, hence under the section Extremities we go through the rubrics to find out what is happening. When we get to Pain which is a sensation we find the first subsection is indeed modality,

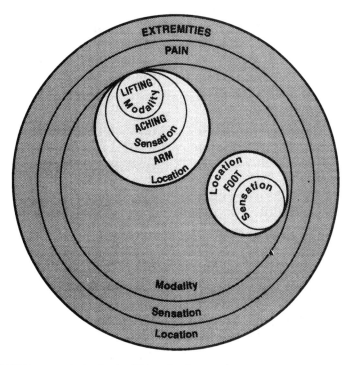

Fig. 11.1 TLSM is repeated wheel within wheel.

then the sublocations follow with their modalities, then more precise sensations of pain, e.g. aching, boring, burning, bursting, cramping, etc. arranged alphabetically. These are then followed by modality, then the location and modality again. There is no need for further location or sensation. Thus arranged diagramatically the order is:

LOCATION   SENSATION   MODALITY
Extremities   Pain   ↓
                        LOCATION → Modality
                        Arm ↓
                        SENSATION → Modality
                        Aching →   Location →   Modality
                                                        Arm   On lifting something

It is appropriate here to put in a note about time and modality, which are often confused because of course time might be a modality, as in '*When* is the arm worse?'. Time is the exciting cause or causation, the point of change. As such it refers more specifically to the vital force, and is found under Generalities. It becomes a modality when it is telling us about the part and what makes the part better or worse. Confusion arises because when the modality is given in the Repertory it starts with time, i.e. morning, 8 a.m., 10 a.m., noon, afternoon, 3 p.m., 4 p.m., evening, etc. Why should a symptom get worse at a specific time? This time phase is a character of the vital force, and not a modality proper. It is in fact a generality, and is an important symptom of individuality. We find it in the Particular section only because it has come to our notice in that context, and is entered here as a clear fact arising in regard to this part.

ACTIVITY 2   Turn to the Extremities section in your Repertory, and find Pain. Go through the entries until you trace the order of recurrence of time, location, sensation and modality.

Kent's Language

Kent uses some language which is unfamiliar to us. In the first instance, he often uses old medical terms which are no longer in use, e.g. the thoracic area of the back he calls the *dorsal* area; he uses the words *nates* to apply to buttocks. There is a further difficulty in that his English is not only over 100 years old, it is also mid-west American. Thus there are subtle differences in usage.

    Kent is otherwise very precise in his use of langauge. It therefore comes as a puzzle to find that in the Mind section he often uses such similar words as sadness, despair and anguish; or anger, rage and irritable. The distinction is obviously one of degree, but it is more than just that: it picks out the finer variations of human emotions. Ortega, the great Mexican homoeopath, states the Kent often uses three entries to express one emotion such as depression, and that each of these entries refer to the emotion as it would be coloured by one of the three miasms. Hence:

Sadness	Psoric	Underfunction
Anguish	Sycotic	Overfunction
Despair	Syphilitic	Destructive, distorting function

Irritable	Psoric	Underfunction
Anger	Sycotic	Overfunction
Rage	Syphilitic	Destructive, distorting function

Putting the rubrics of the Mind section under these three headings certainly gives one a greater understanding of Kent's language.

The Other Repertories

The other repertories can be found in a scale somewhere between Phatak and Kent in their ordering system. None are as complete as Kent's Repertory. Boericke's is similar to Phatak's in containing a great deal of common use and clinical headings, but it is organized in sections like Kent's. Boericke is commonly found in use among the laity, because it also contains a short but full Materia Medica, very similar to Phatak's Materia Medica but much more concise.

Boenninghausen's Repertory is seldom used except for his 'sides of the body' and Remedy Relationships, often incorporated as an appendix to some editions of Kent's Repertory. Gibson incorporated his Remedy Relationships into a table, often also appended to Kent's Repertory.

Most Repertories, such as Clarke's and Farringdon's, are based on their studies of Materia Medica. Clarke is useful in his own right, as mentioned previously, because of its useful section on causation.

Hering's *Analytical Repertory of the Mind* is useful in approaching the Kent style of Materia Medica study, in which mental and emotional symptoms are stressed

Yet other Repertories, such as *The Synthetic Repertory*, either try to bring in more modern findings of Materia Medica or simply look at the organization of the rubrics from slightly different angles. In modern days there are also computer Repertory systems. The most complete, based on Kent's Repertory, would appear to be the *Mac Repertory* produced by Roger Morrison and Bill Gray.

ACTIVITY 3 List the different types of pain found under the head, Pain, section, e.g. burning, darting.

ACTIVITY 4 How many different areas of the abdomen are listed under Abdomen, Pain?
List them, then draw a diagram of the abdomen labelling where they are to be found. You can check this in any anatomy and physiology textbook.

ACTIVITY 5 Unless you have medical experience there are some areas of human symptoms of which you have no experience, which people seldom talk about and unfortunately will not volunteer, so you must have some idea of the variety in order to gently coax such symptoms from the patient! You may thus benefit from studying the following categories in the Repertory.

Stool
Urine
Vomit
Expectoration
Vision
Hearing
Chill
Fever
And Others

Many of these are objective symptoms, of which you should be able to get an accurate description either from the patient or your own observations.

ACTIVITY 6 The following symptoms occur under the Mind section of the Repertory. Put them into words that the patient of today might use to denote that symptom.

Chagrin
Anticipation
Forsaking
Exaltation of fancy
Mania a Potou

Anxiety of conscience
Theorizing
Inconstancy
Grimaces
Starting
Monomania
Malicious

ACTIVITY 7 The following symptoms are used by patients today to describe mental states. Under what rubric would these be found in the Repertory?

Agoraphobia
Indecisive
Suicidal
Grumbling all the time
Randy
Spends much time on his own thinking of things
Perfectionist
Frantic
Can't face work
On the go all the time
Does not know what he wants
Fear of choking

ACTIVITY 8 Find the page number in Kent's Repertory of the following symptoms.

Pain behind the ear, better in the open air
A crack down the middle of the tongue
Pustular eruptions on the right side of the abdomen
Pain in the region of the umbilicus
Palpitations at 3 a.m.
Hand itchy after rubbing
Partial paralysis of the foot
Patient worse from brandy consumption
Sensation of fullness in the head
Pain in the eye as if from sand
Painless ulcers on the lower lip
Empty sensations in the stomach during nausea
Abdominal pain as if squeezed between two stones
Bowel movements olive green
Fear of pins
Sensitive to the slightest noise
Aversion to her own sex
Moist eruption on the head
Eyes dry on reading
Nose bleeding from right side
Burning heat on the upper lip
Lower jaw twitches
Constant inclination to clench the teeth together
Discharge from the back of the nose
Nausea during headache
Cancer of the ovaries
Bloody discharge after menstruation
Sensation of a plug in the larynx
Racking cough at night

Sensation as if a weight on the chest
Swelling of the axillary glands
Pain in the back with desire to urinate
Cold hands during fever
Dark redness of tonsils
Sleep disturbed by dreams
Patient worse taking butter
Fatigue after eating

ACTIVITY 9

Find some examples in your friends and relatives.
Describe the symptoms as clearly as you can, then attempt to find the symptoms in the Repertory, e.g.

Gran's rheumatism.
Your daughter's earache.
Your husband's/wife's depression.
Your son's wart.
Your roommate's PMT.

Remember to complete the symptom according to TLSM.

If possible, find general symptoms too,
e.g. when does this person generally feel low?

ACTIVITY 10

Here are some more symptoms to look up in the Repertory.
The more you familiarize yourself with this book, the better it will serve you and your patients.

Find the page number and note if the symptom is strange, rare and peculiar, general, mental and emotional, or particular.

Numbness in the forearm in the morning
Pulsation deep in the inguinal region
Falling backwards during convulsions
Skin itches when walking in the open air
Nausea on waking
Greedy for money and possessions
Mucus membrane of the mouth discoloured blue
Dizzy and nauseous
Feels rejected
Worse after eating pork
Low back pain as if crushed
Hawks up hard mucus plugs
Worse after taking the clothes off
Wounds heal slowly
Urine smells sweet
Sensation of a lump rising in the throat
Jaws clenched
Objects seem too large
Unable to keep the eyes open
Cannot make up his mind about anything
Laughs constantly
The head feels empty when talking
Feels knotted inside
Wrings the hands and gesticulates

Lump in the left breast
Stitching pain in the armpit
Wakes before midnight
Symptoms aggravated from sweating
Everything feels unreal
No feelings or sensations on the skin

READINGS

Vithoulkas G *The science of homoeopathy*, Ch. 14

Repertorization 1

Headings: What is Repertorization?
Drawbacks
The Process of Repertorization
Examples
Summary of Practice Points

Aim: By the end of this lesson you should be able to look up symptoms of a case in Kent's Repertory and isolate a few remedies that cover the total symptom picture. The skills involved here entail a great deal of practice, and assimilation of the next two lessons.

What is Repertorization?

The Repertory is a very valuable resource that puts together all the symptoms produced in provings. Under each symptom are found all the remedies that produce that symptom in the provings. Since there are over 2000 remedies, and we cannot know them all or even remember *all* the symptoms of each, this is a valuable aide memoire.

The process of repertorization therefore enables us to bring together a list of remedies that produce all the symptoms that appear in a case. This provides a selection from which we can choose the best-fit remedy. This choice is made not on the repertorization process, but on our knowledge of:

- Philosophy
- Materia Medica
- The patient's pattern of disease.

Drawbacks to Repertorization

There are several ways in which the Repertory may let us down, and there are several ways in which we can abuse it – usually by using it too woodenly. The Repertory does not always contain the experiences of today's patients, so we must select carefully the words used to describe the symptoms. The next lesson will look at this problem in more detail. Once we have the right language there are still two problems.

Quantitative

There is a limit to the data actually present in the Repertory.

- Many sensations and strange, rare and peculiar symptoms are not present in the Repertory. H. A. Roberts little book *Sensations as If . . .* is thus a valuable companion to the Repertory.
- Some provings have not yet been added to the Repertory in print.
- Some remedies are still poorly proved today and hence are poorly represented in the Repertory. This applies in particular to 'minor remedies'.
- Major polycrests such as Thuja, Tuberculinum and Natrum Muriaticum are poorly represented in the Repertory.
- Many nosodes are not included in the Repertory. There are no bowel nosodes, no Carcinosins, Pertussin, Morbillinum, Rubella, X-Ray, Folliculinum, Cortizone, Influenzinum, etc.
- Many modern substances to which patients are exposed have not been proved, and are therefore not included in the Repertory: E numbers, monosodium glutamate, plastic and various alloys. Thus when there is a possibility that these are maintaining causes it is difficult to isolate and identify them.

Qualitative

Qualitative criticism of the Repertory is more serious than quantitative. Most of the provings from which the Repertory draws are not based on the Vithoulkas mode, which seeks out the subtle pure reactions of the remedy. Old-style provings produce a broad band of symptoms like a bell curve (Fig. 12.1). The criteria along this curve show the relationship between susceptibility and the type of symptoms produced. Those more sensitive to the remedies produce rarer symptoms, which form a small percentage at one end of the curve, whereas those most commonly produced, and thus characteristic of the remedy, are in the centre or the highest point of the bell-shaped curve, and are printed in bold type in the Repertory. At the other end of the curve, in plain type, are symptoms produced by just a few provers. Often these are physical symptoms peculiar to the prover's own symptom picture. These less important symptoms may not be highly significant in the remedy, but they have the same grade of type as the more important S, R & P symptoms. Strange, rare and peculiar symptoms are recorded in the Repertory in ordinary type because so few provers were sensitive enough to that remedy to produce them.

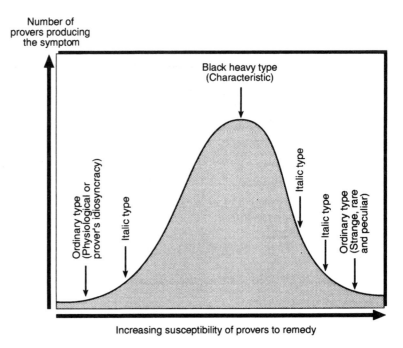

Fig. 12.1   Increasing susceptibility of provers to remedy.

When we look at the repertorization process you will see that most attention and credence is given to remedies that appear in bold type. These are characteristic symptoms, but we are looking for that which is unique and individual. These words individual and characteristic have appeared again, and since there is a contradiction I am anxious for you to know the difference: individual means unique, and that is what we prescribe on, but we use characteristic to identify a person's type, and this involves rounding off their attributes into common patterns. The Repertory helps us to characterize but our knowledge of Materia Medica helps us to individualize, and gives us a better perspective (see Lesson 14). Some individual aspects of the case may be lost when we rely on the most commonly occurring symptoms! The repertorization process tends to round off the symptom picture to produce polycrest remedies in the main. It is even possible, when using elimination techniques of repertorization, to lose the indicative remedy! We will look at this in more detail later.

THE MOST COMMON WAY TO LOSE THE REMEDY IS THROUGH INCORRECT INTERPRETATION OF DATA OR THROUGH INSUFFICIENT DATA. Examples will appear in this and the next two lessons.

The Process of Repertorization

There are seven steps:

1)   Select prescribing symptoms from your collected data (see Lesson 14).

2) Describe the prescribing symptoms in the language of the repertory.
3) Organize the prescribing symptoms into a hierarchy of symptoms.
4) Using first the mental and emotional symptoms, collect all those remedies that appear under the most important rubrics.
5) Collect all those remedies that appear under the general symptoms that also relate to the mental and emotional symptoms.
6) Use the most individual particular symptoms to further differentiate between remedies.
7) Refer to the Materia Medica.

This process is based on the assumption that a well proven remedy will produce its most characteristic symptoms very highly marked in the provers, and that these will then be highly marked in the listing in the Repertory. Of course they must also be highly marked in the patient, and this is why you have chosen them as prescribing symptoms.

Summary of 1, 2 and 3   Select those symptoms most individual to the case. Put them in the language of the Repertory so you can look them up (Lesson 11), and finally organize them into a hierarchy as you were taught in Lesson 4.

PRACTICE POINT   You have already found that there is more than one interpretation of a symptom, so in practice make sure you have clearly determined the meaning before approaching this stage – preferably during case-taking.

Selecting Prescribing Symptoms   The greatest of care must be exercised when symptoms are selected, as the choice already discounts most of our remedies. Thus, if the patient is angry when contradicted, and is seen to be very impatient, we need not consider any remedies that do not occur under these two rubrics as, however else we describe the patient, he or she must be labelled as *angry when contradicted* and *very impatient*.

PRACTICE POINT   Thus also, one of the first things we check when we are not satisfied with the outcome of the remedy is the selection of the correct prescribing symptoms, and the most precise language to express these in Repertory terms.

Mental and Emotional Symptoms   In his essay at the beginning of most editions of the Repertory, Kent suggests that the highest grade of symptom should be strong feelings – hate, desire, aversions of a mental type – and that these should be followed by symptoms of the intellect, then by symptoms of the memory.

The emotional components of mental experience thus come first because of the amount of energy represented. Examples are anger, grief, excitement, vexation, disappointed love, etc. Note that these are dysfunctions of the normal emotional state.

Mental level dysfunctions are insanities, neuroses and psychoses, which have more importance than the emotions unless intensity of the other decrees otherwise. Other aspects of the mental level, changes in consciousness such as epilepsy and aphasia, are determined by physiological dysfunction of the brain, and so are less important and may even be relegated to the particulars as dysfunctions of the brain as an organ. What is left of the mental level forms the temperament or personality, or mind. Whatever mind is, it is a highly evolved and complex process unique to humans. Robert Davidson helps us to put it into the language of the Repertory when he divides it into three faculties: will, understanding and memory.

Will he describes as the active, expressive side: 'I express', which shows malfunction in disturbances of social instinct, affectations, phobias, life preservation (suicide, loathing of life, murderousness, violence) loves, hates, fears, etc.

Understanding is described as the passive side of the mental faculties, involving imagination, intellect (as we would use that term today, meaning cognitive skills), delusions, dreams, sense of proportion, clarity of ideas or lack of them, idiocy, etc.: 'I interpret'.

Memory is the last mental symptom in order of importance, and involves concentration, weakness or lack of memory, mistakes in reading, writing, speaking, etc.

Since today's patients would appear to have more mental complexity than in Kent's day, this expansion of Kent's theme is to be welcomed.

The mental and emotional symptoms come after the S, R & P symptoms in the hierarchy. When you look up the symptom in the Repertory you now copy down all the remedies that appear under that rubric; but there are over 100 remedies that appear under the rubric 'anger'. This is a key to the fact that the symptom is not very useful, and we should remember Kent's comments about 'pages and pages of symptoms'. It should cause us to look for a better prescribing symptom, symptoms that stop and make use hesitate, i.e. that are more individual. There are no easy rules here. The skills involved in selecting good prescribing symptoms are learned through day-to-day contact with such data, and with the work of the practitioner in the clinic, and through classroom discussion within a group – this is where the lone student is handicapped. Hopefully the examples used in this lesson and in the next two will help start the process.

How do you put aside your own prejudice to objectively assess mental and emotional symptoms? How do you label subjective symptoms with the precision required? Is it important if someone is angry, or that his boss was outrageous, or that he was more sensitive today because his hair is greasy and it frustrates him? Were things really simpler in Kent's day? The homoeopath is a very skilled person. Clinical training teaches objectivity, and case analysis enables us to look more deeply into human nature. This comes with experience and is one of the benefits of working with a skilled practitioner during clinical training.

General Symptoms

Only when the mental reaction is covered and the case reduced to ten or so remedies does Kent approach the generals. This is of course very sound advice indeed, coming from a master. If your general symptoms are well selected you can now use them to reduce the number of remedies you found under the mental and emotional symptoms.

Particular Symptoms

You should now have a select group of maybe 10–20 remedies. You may have even less. To reduce these further, select the most individual particular symptoms and then isolate those remedies that occur under these particular rubrics.

There is a difficulty here, however: Kent's Repertory has been criticized as having rubrics that are either too large or too small – so large that the practitioner was handing hundreds of remedies rather than ten or so, or so small that there is not enough to choose from. When we get down to the level of particular symptoms it is easy to go astray. Many remedies have not been proved down to this level, and so they are not represented in the Repertory.

Look up the Materia Medica

You should now have just a few remedies. To further decide between these you must go over the whole case again, comparing it with the Materia Medica. Have you fully understood the case? Does a theme or essence run all the way through each symptom, and is this expressed in one of the remedies that you have now selected?

PRACTICE POINT

If your repertorization does not produce a little group of remedies, then look at your data again. Are your prescribing symptoms startling enough to make you hesitate?
If there is no individuality in your case, go back to your patient and find it.
If you have good information, did you translate it into the language of the Repertory with accuracy?

With greater accuracy in mind there is no harm whatever in going back over the case anyway, to check that the theme or essence of the remedy you have chosen runs through all the symptoms, and that there is a cohesive coherent total symptom picture.

Once again I say, there is great skill in hearing the patient and in translating his or her idiom into the language of the Materia Medica. There is skill in understanding what exactly the patient means. Perhaps I have said it often enough to make you realize that these are the two areas that give rise to the greatest number of mistakes, and you must start the process with sound data, good case-taking. Without this, repertorization can be very misleading. Let us look at some cases and put some of these observations to work.

Example 1

Female aged 8 years.
Flies into a rage when the accident is mentioned.
Introverted since the accident which she thinks she caused.
Hides behind mother when a stranger is present.
Fatigued.
Chilly.
Sucks thumb.
Blonde hair.

The order above is that in which these symptoms were placed during the exercise in Lesson 4. The most recent symptoms are put first, showing us the most recent and, as in this case, often the most intensive disturbance. From the third symptom down the symptoms refer to the constitutional picture rather than as a result of the accident.

The Mental and Emotional Symptoms

From the evidence given, guilt is implied because the child's behaviour has changed since the accident. The key phrase above is 'which she thinks she caused', especially when she reacts so strongly when the subject is mentioned. Despite my comments in Lesson 4, I have used the rubric guilt to simplify the repertorization.

Guilt is found in the Repertory as 'Anxiety of conscience', which has 41 remedies. Rage is a much larger rubric, but note that whereas guilt can be determined objectively from the patient's behaviour, rage is a judgement of the intensity of the anger.

How do we look up 'Hides behind mother on entering the room in the presence of a stranger'. It may be a desire to hide,

- Aggravated in the presence of a stranger,
- or is it just
- Timidity?

Despite the comments on the last two symptoms it looks as if we have a good case with some individuality expressed. Let us see how it repertorizes:

Guilt   **alum, am.c, ars, aur**, cact, canth, carb.s, *carb.v, caust,* **chel**, cina, *cocc*, coff, *con*, cupr, cycl, **dig**, *ferr*, fer.ar, ferr.p, **graph**, hyos, *ign*, mag.s, *medd, merc, nat.m*, nit.ac, *nux.v*, phos, **psor**, puls, rheum, *rhus.t*, ruta, sabad, *sil*, stront, *sulph, thuj, verat, zinc.*

Of these remedies only the following appear under **rage**, but whatever remedy the patient needs it must contain **guilt**:

Rage   *ars,* **canth***, carb.s*, chel, cina, *cupr*, dig, graph, **hyos***, merc*, nat m, *nit.*ac, *phos*, ruta, sabad, *sulph*, verat, zinc.

Now the list of possible remedies has been cut down because, whatever the best-fit remedy, it must contain **rage**, but this is a child. How important is **rage** when this individual has so little experience, and therefore avenues to express such an overwhelming emotion?

When I took the next M/E symptom I went back to the first rubric so as not to miss anything. There was a doubt about which language to use to express the next symptom, so I looked up all of them:

Desires to hide   ars, cupr, hyos, puls.
Agg in the presence   con, *thuj.*
of a stranger
Bashful   aur, carb v, con, coff, *cupr*, hyos, *ign*,
                  merc, nit.ac, nux.v, phos, **puls**, *sulph*,
                  zinc.

As you can see, whatever rubric I choose will automatically alter the outcome, so can I use any of them? I must have clear facts before I make a choice.

Generalities

There is one more rubric to view: **chilly**, which is a general found in the Repertory under **Lack of vital heat**:

Lack of vital heat   *alum, am.c*, **ars**, aur, cact, *carb s, carb v*,
                  caust, *chel, cocc, con, dig*, **ferr, graph**,
                  medd, merc, nat.m, **nit.ac**, nux.v, **phos,**
                  psor, rhus t, *sabad*, **sil**, *stront, sulph, thuj*,
                  zinc.

Analysis

There are still far too many remedies from which to make a choice. The problem belongs in the case-taking, which was not precise enough. However, if for practice purposes we were to assume that **bashful** were the right rubric, then, including the general symptom, we would be down to ten remedies, namely:

aur, carb.v, con, cupr, hyos, merc, nit.ac, nux v, phos, zinc.

If we could add **rage**, this would leave only four remedies:

merc, nit ac, phos, sulph.

Had we been sure of our symptoms, we would turn to the Materia Medica at this stage. As things stand, we do not have a case.

Example 2

Female, aged 34 years.
Sweats on the face while eating.
Weeps without cause.
Thirst for large quantities.
Worse fasting.
Worse for cold food and drink.
Worse before menses.
Constipation, dry hard stools.
Back pain < lifting
            < rubbing
            < heat.

Strange, Rare and Peculiar (S, R & P)

The first symptom is S, R & P, and quickly reduces the number of remedies:

Face, perspiration while eating *ign, nat.m, sulph.*

Although I note this symptom, I put it aside as narrowing down the field too quickly, especially when teaching students. If one of these remedies is required, it will not be lost by proceeding as before but starting with the next symptom. In fact, we will have a control with which to test the result.

Mental and Emotional

Weeping without cause Apis, ars, bell, camph, *cina, graph,* hura, kali.ar, kali.br, kali.c, kreos, *lyc, nat.m,* nit.ac, **puls**, staph, **sulph**, tarent, viol.o, *zinc.*

Now we have a better state of affairs, starting from a good mental and emotional symptom. Now, let us add a few generals.

Generalities

Worse fasting ars, cina, *graph*, ign, kali.c, kreos, lyc, nit.ac, puls, **staph**, *sulph.*

Note that we have taken only those remedies that appear under the rubric **weeping without cause**. If this M/E symptom truly represents the patient, then whichever remedy is needed must be represented under this rubric, so it is unnecessary to consider others. However, the quick-witted among you will realize that I have added **ignatia**, which was eliminated under **weeping without cause**. This is both pedantic and superstitious on my part, because I want to check the occurrence of all three remedies that appeared under the S, R & P rubric **Face, perspiration while eating**.

Let us consider some more generals:

Worse cold food   **ars**, *graph*, ign, kali.ar, *kali.c*, kreos, **lyc**, nat.m, nit.ac, *puls, sulph.*

Worse cold drink   apis, *bell, graph, ign*, kali.ar, kali.c, *lyc*, puls, *sulph, tarent.*

Worse before menses   bell, graph, lyc, *kali.c, kreos,* **lyc, nat.m, puls**, staph, **sulph, zinc.**

Thirst for large quantities   ars, camph, **nat.m, sulph.**

Now, this case is very different from Example 1. The language is precise. There is even one remedy that goes through all the rubrics – through the strange, rare and peculiar, the mental and emotional symptoms, and the generals.

Note that I displaced **Thirst for large quantities** as the rubric was too small. Also, I did not eliminate remedies as I stepped down through the hierarchy. The repertory is my tool to enable a wider choice. The final selection of the remedy depends on knowledge of Materia Medica, so there is nothing to lose by considering a few extra remedies, especially when the numbers dealt with are so small. On the plus side, this is a useful way of studying Materia Medica comparison.

Had I progressively eliminated, I would have got the following:

- **Face, perspiration while eating** *ign, nat.m, sulph.*
- **Weeping without cause**   *nat.m,* **sulph.**
- **Thirst for large quantities**   **nat.m, sulph.**
- **Worse fasting**   *sulph*
- **Worse cold food**   *sulph*
- **Worse cold drink**   *sulph*
- **Worse before menses**   **sulph**

However, in order to justify the choice of **sulphuricum** it should be seen to cover the particulars, and this is a further check on its validity.

Particulars

Stool dry   ars, kali.ar, kali.c, **lyc, nat.m, nit.ac,** puls, staph, *sulph, zinc.*

Stool hard   *ars, kali.ar, kali.c,* kreos, **lyc, nat.m, nit ac**, *puls*, staph, **sulph, zinc.**

99

The hard dry stool is not contained in a single rubric, but in two. When this happens, the two rubrics can be added together because the stool is not hard *or* dry but hard *and* dry. As it is, the only difference between the remedies occurring under the two rubrics in this case is qualitative. **Sulphuricum** is still well represented.

Back pain better rubbing	puls
Worse lifting	**graph, lyc**
Better heat	*ars, bell*, hyos, ign, lyc, *nat.m*, puls, zinc.

The back pain modalities contain no **sulphuricum** whatever. Does this then discount **sulphuricum** as the remedy? The rubrics are very small. If we go back to the Generalities section to look up the modalities, we will find the rubrics are larger and produce more interesting results.

As the symptoms are represented here, the modalities are attached to particular symptoms but it is possible that this is the general way in which this patient expresses illness of this type! In this case there are not enough disordered particulars to show the general nature of the modalities. Personally, I am not happy to use a general modality for a particular symptom, although in this case I can make an exception because it is the last symptom and all else fits well.

Analysis

Ignatia comes through all the symptoms of the generalities but it does not come through the mental and emotional symptoms, or the symptoms of the stool.

Natrum Muriaticum is well represented at all levels, but tends to dart in and out of the symptoms, being absent from many.

Are there any other remedies that are not represented in the strange, rare and peculiar that come through all the other symptoms?

Lycopodium is very well represented, except in better for rubbing. **Zinc** is well represented at all levels, but like **Natrum Muriaticum** it disappears in some symptoms. **Pulsatilla** comes through all the generals and the mental and emotionals, and is represented in the stool symptoms and in the back symptoms that were repertorized under particulars. **Arsenicum** is well represented at all levels but, like **Natrum Muriaticum** and **Zinc**, disappears from some symptoms.

This also applies to **Graphites, Cina, Arsenicum** and **Kali Carbonicum**, and to **Kreosotium** and **Nitric acid**. We could make a good case for **Sulphuricum**, but **Sulphuricum** is notoriously **Worse heat** generally.

Under the rubric **Heat** in Generalities, nothing fits this context. **Warm** is another rubric under Generalities which is more appropriate when heat is external. However, even here there is no rubric that covers **Better warm applications** – *most* conditions are better for warm applications.

Now look under **Cold**: 'cold in general aggravates' is the opposite of 'heat aggravates', but could be the same as 'warm applications ameliorate'?? Under this section we find **Sulphuricum** again. So, **Sulphuricum** is the only remedy which could be covered by *all* the rubrics.

Example 3

Female aged 26.
Epistaxis when menses are absent.
Black blood in long threads.
Numbness right side.
Anxiety prevents sleep.
Anger before lunch.
Dissatisfaction *re* job.
Nausea in the evening.

Strange, Rare and Peculiar (S, R & P)

The first two symptoms are strange, rare and peculiar, but as in Example 2, the strange, rare and peculiar symptom is too unique to produce many remedies.

Epistaxis, menses absent *bry, graph, cham, lach.*

To find black blood in long threads we must add two rubrics together:

Nose, Epistaxis, dark blood bapt, **croc** *kali. bi*, mag. c, *merc*, **sec**, *sep.*
Nose, Epistaxis stringy blood bapt, **croc**, *cupr, kali. bi*, mag. c, *merc*, **sec**, *sep.*

Note that these remedies are entirely different from those in **Epistaxis, menses absent**. This is a warning that something is not right. First, we check that the language is correct: epistaxis instead of menses is also called, more correctly, **Vicarious menstruation**. This rubric is found under Genitalia Female, and has a larger group of remedies:

acon, ars, bapt, bell, **bry**, cact. *calc*, chin,
cimic, coll, *crot.h, dig*, dulc, ferr, *ham*, mill, nux v, **phos**, puls, *sang, senec*,
sep, sulph, ust, zinc.

Referring specifically to bleeding from the nose, we can also look under Nose, Epistaxis, Vicarious, but this contains only five remedies:

bry, **cham**, *lach*, **phos**, *puls.*

Black blood in long threads is actually a keynote that would point to only a few remedies. However, there is no rubric containing it in the repertory. Two of these remedies, **Bryonia** and **Lachesis**, occur under **Vicarious menstruation**, or even **Vicarious epistaxis**, but neither is contained under **Stringy haemorrhage from the nose**. Only **Baptisia** and **Sepia** are found under both. The rubric **Vicarious menstruation** or **Epistaxis** is very objective, whereas **Black blood in long threads** is subjective. When is blood black, dark, or dark red? Get your friends to describe a few colours to you. And long threads . . .? Is this the same as stringy? Could it be described as mucous? How long do the threads have to be – a few inches or over a foot? The last is not so ludicrous as it sounds after you have spoken to a few patients.

Let us look at the next strange, rare and peculiar symptom to see if we can get any further forward. This is also a general symptom, which is to be found under Generalities as a **Numbness**. To add **Rightsidedness**, in this case, we must combine **Right-sided**, also to be found under Generalities thus:

Numbness	*acon, ars, bapt, bell*, **bry**, cact, calc, chin, cimic, *crot.h*, dig, dulc, ferr, *nux v*, **phos**, *puls, sep*, sulph, *zinc*.
Right-sided	*acon*, **ars, bapt, bell, bry, calc**, chin, **crot.h**, dulc, **nux v, puls**, *sulph, zinc*.

At this point, **Sepia, Lachesis** and **Phosphoricum** are eliminated, as they are distinctly left-sided remedies. From our Materia Medica, we know how left-sided they are so we let them go. We might have been more reluctant if it were only a part which was right-sided, but here it is a general symptom.

Mental and Emotional

Anxiety before sleep contains some of our remedies. **Anxiety on going to sleep** contains **Aconite** and **Pulsatilla** only.

The Generality **Worse before sleeping** is a much larger rubric. After all, anxiety is perhaps the largest rubric in the Repertory, and is thus insignificant were it not for the modality, that the patient is anxious **before sleep**:

Worse before sleep acon, ars, *bell*, **bry, calc**, *chin*, dulc, nux v, **puls, sulph**, zinc.

Now we have also lost **Baptisia**, leaving only **Bryonia** from the remedies for **Black blood in long threads**.

Dissatisfied (Discontented in the Repertory) acon, *ars, bry*, calc, *chin*, dulc, *nux v, puls*, **sulph**.

There are still a lot of remedies possible, so let us look at the generals.

General Symptoms

There is only one general symptom:

Nausea in the Evening bapt, bry, *calc*, nux v, *puls*, sulph.

This does not get us very far. Baptisia is the only remedy which is pushed out by this rubric, and it is also pushed out in the rubric Dissatisfied.

Analysis

If we put all three of the last rubrics together, then only five remedies remain: **Bryonia, Calcarea, Nux vomica, Pulsatilla, Sulphuricum**.

How do we tell the difference between these five when we have no more symptoms? The Materia Medica tells us Bryonia is the remedy, since it has the keynotes. Such a choice would be sound enough in the absence of other evidence. However, there is another way that is sometimes appropriate.

The appearance of each remedy under a rubric is given a number of points, thus a remedy in bold type is worth three points, one in italics is worth two points, and one in ordinary type is worth one point. Thus if we count the total number of occurrences we get:

Bryonia	15
Calc	12
Nux vomica	10
Pulsatilla	15 (17 if we include anxiety before sleep)
Sulphur	11

If we also add the number of rubrics each appears under, then we get the following:

Bryonia	7
Calc	6
Nux vomica	6
Pulsatilla	8 (if we include anxiety before sleep)
Sulphur	6

In this case the number of rubrics adds little to the points. However, now **Pulsatilla** comes forward as worthy of consideration before all others: quantity suggests **Pulsatilla** as the right selection, but knowledge of the Materia Medica still says **Bryonia** is the choice, because **Black blood in long threads** is a strange, rare and peculiar symptom of **Bryonia**. So **Bryonia** is given.

Summary of Practice Points

1) Make sure you have clearly determined the meaning of the symptoms before organizing them into a hierarchy.
2) If not satisfied with the outcome of the remedy, check that the correct prescribing symptoms have been selected and that they are expressed in the most precise language possible.
3) If your repertorization does not produce a little group of remedies, then re-examine your data.

ACTIVITY 1

Now to learn more you should try a little of this yourself. Finish the other seven cases in Lesson 4, and there are another ten cases added to this lesson. Note that the cases are too small to suggest a 'right' answer. The object of the exercise is to familiarize yourself with the process of repertorization.

ADDITIONAL CASES

1) Forgetful, better in the morning. Urine dark and scanty. Desires highly seasoned food. Sweats only on left side. Cracked nipples. Ulcers on the foot. Desires cold drinks. Hair falling. Menses too early. Warts on fingers. Nymphomania.

2) Vertigo, sensation of ascending. Stiffness in the cervical areas. Worse after sitting. Flushes of heat upwards. Early, scanty and prolonged menses. Palpitations in the evening, and in bed. Corns and chilblains on the toes. Vivid dreams of an amorous nature. Laughs at serious things. Irritable at noise. Cyst left breast. Skin burns and stings, better scratching. Desires company and aggravated when alone.

3) Emphysema, cough worse 3–4 a.m. Dry cough with many colds. Weeps easily, especially in the morning. Menses absent, or as if would appear. Leucorrhoea offensive. Dread of bath. Bathing affected parts ameliorates. Right foot numb. Cramp in calves. Overweight. Desires open air.

4) Eczema around joints since childhood. Asthma 3–4 a.m., worse physical exertion, better sleep. Wakes 4 a.m. cannot return to sleep. Desires sour food. Fear of the dark. Fastidious. Shakes during sleep. Walks in sleep occasionally. Underweight.

5) Eczema better in winter, better abroad. Gets other children to scratch her knees for her. Likes to be occupied. Needs attention all the time. Dislikes to eat in the morning. Wakes 3 a.m. Dreams of falling.

6) Abdominal pain, epigastric, worse for tight clothing. Flatulence. Anxiety about health. Sarcastic. Irritable on exposure to noise. Works as a photographer, could have been big in films. Eats only rice. High blood pressure. Frightful dreams of dogs. Skin burns on parts lain on.

7) Cramps in calves at night. Headaches with nausea on Sunday. Sense of heat on top of head. Weeps at night without cause. Desires fresh air. Worse in the morning generally. Wakes screaming at 3 a.m. Sudden urge to urinate. Stiffness of the neck. Desires sweets and highly seasoned food. Vertigo causing to fall to the left.

8) Psoriasis all over, much itching, better heat, better sun. History of bronchitis. Aggressive. Restless. Concentration poor. Ravenous appetite. Much heat. Easily excited. Fastidious. Granular eyelids, worse bathing.

9) Craves curries and highly seasoned foods. Loves garlic. Untidy. Jealous and flies into a rage when partner flirts at parties. Vertigo in high places. Likes company. Changes job frequently. Hates the cold and loves the heat. Desires salt. Desires alcohol. Dreams of work. Sleepy in the afternoon and after food. Waterbrash. White discharge. Loss of interest in sex of late.

10) Eyes have a glassy appearance. Green discharge from the nose. Complaints started 3 years ago when Gran died. Indifferent to work. Irritable after eating. Cold extremities.

READINGS

The following four essays are usually found at the beginning of most editions of the Repertory.

Kent J T *Use of the Repertory*
       How to Study the Repertory
       How to use the Repertory
Tyler M, Weir J *Repertorising*

ADDITIONAL READING

Kent J T *1986 Repertory of homoeopathic materia medica.* Jain, New Delhi
Tyler M *Different ways of finding the remedy.* World Homoeopathic, New Delhi

LESSON THIRTEEN

Repertorization 2

Headings: The Language of the Patient
Case Example

Aim: In this lesson we will explore the difference between the language of the Repertory and the language of the patient, and emphasize the importance of exact interpretation of the patient's language.

Objectives: To be able put the patient's symptoms into the appropriate language of the Materia Medica.

The Language of the Patient

In previous exercises I have selected the symptoms and put them into the language of the Materia Medica for you. Now, I want to show you how to make the transition yourself. The patient's description of his or her symptoms, and other evidence from case taking, will be labelled raw data, because it has not yet been interpreted or analysed.

The Words Used

The language of the Materia Medica is the prover's description of his or her symptoms. This was simple language at the time the proving symptoms were collected. It is difficult for us today for two reasons:

Language use has changed a great deal over a century;
Our environment and experiences have also changed.

Much of the Materia Medica contains objective descriptions for which each person may use slightly different wording, depending on his or her own experience and bias. When taking the case the practitioner needs to feel and sense the patient's meaning, and then find the most appropriate rubric in the Repertory to express this meaning. For example, throbbing is described in the Repertory as *pulsating*. Other terms used by the patient might be thumping, pounding, like hammers.

The Structure and Function of Language

Part of language is its structure and meaning. Words can be organized in different ways; language can be factual, hypothetical, opinionated, vague or suggestive. In the example below, the prescribing symptoms of the penis are objective and clear. The information about the patient's childhood is part opinion. What happened in his first relationship is unknown. Any statement we might make on this outside of his statement of distress would be hypothetical. His statement that 'he would like to visit friends but feels lost and can't get it together' is vague, but it is easy to trip ahead with suppositions or theories. *YOU MUST NOT.*

You must clarify the data when taking the case. There is therefore a skill in case-taking to check the data for quality as you receive it.

Let us look at a short case, pick out the prescribing symptoms and study the effect of different choices of words on finding the remedy.

Case Example

Raw Data

The patient, a 25-year-old man, suffers inflammation at the tip of the penis, which is red and sore. As a child he was bullied at school, even in the sixth form. He thinks it was because he was smaller than others, that others took advantage of him. Although he was very angry, he did nothing about the bullying. He now finds it difficult to tell people he likes them because he fears rejection. He is unhappy at present regarding his girlfriend. He feels he would like more security and he would like to settle down and perhaps have children. The penis symptoms have been there off and on since his first sexual encounter years ago. His was very distressed when this relationship ended. He is a jealous person. He has a great deal of anger at his situation and yet is very sad, even grieved, and a bit on edge lest his feelings erupt and the girlfriend rejects him. He cannot face the future by himself. He would like to go away and visit friends but feels lost and cannot get it together. The penis symptoms are worse after intercourse and masturbation. There is burning when he urinates.

Prescribing Symptoms

The first step is to select those symptoms that must be cured by the remedy, *the prescribing symptoms*. These must then be converted into appropriate language.

ACTIVITY 1 　　Before we look at these, make your own selection.

What is wrong with this patient?
What makes you stop and hesitate?

The presenting symptom in this case is the inflammation of the penis. There is little need to find other language as the above is simple and descriptive. Hence the prescribing symptoms are as follows:

Section (of Rep.)	Rubric	T, L, S, M	Further detail/Remarks
Genitalia (Male)	Inflammation	Penis (glans) tip of	Glans
	Pain	Sore	
	Redness	Glans	

'He finds it difficult to tell people he likes them because he fears rejection'. This is the first statement of fact after the presenting symptoms. What comes before is opinion and therefore open to too many possible interpretations. We can learn little from such speculations.

The next symptom is 'unhappiness regarding his girlfriend'; although this is clear, what does it tell you? He is sad. This is a rubric in the Mind section.

'He would like security, to settle down and have children'. How many different ways could this be interpreted? Do not speculate.

'The penis symptoms have been there on and off since his first sexual encounter 7 years ago'. This is an exciting cause of the penis symptoms, but what is the symptom? 'He was very distressed when the relationship ended'. Is there something here that I can look up in the Repertory? **Disappointed love, Remorse, Anxiety of conscience** . . . ? How can you choose any of these? What facts are actually known to you?

He says he is 'jealous', has a great deal of 'anger', 'sadness', even 'grief', and is on edge *lest his feelings erupt and the girlfriend rejects him*'. There are a number of symptoms here and I do not want to pre-empt the next lesson on case analysis. Thus let us take the data as given, looking at different ways these are expressed in the Repertory.

We also have: 'He cannot face the future by himself' – is this **Fear to be alone, Fear of the future** or **Fear of being deserted**? When taking the case, you must clarify this with the patient. The difficulty here is not in finding the rubric in the Repertory. As it stands, the symptom is not clear enough to use – it is vague.

The penis symptoms are 'worse after intercourse, worse masturbation'. These are straightforward modalities, the sense is clear. The word intercouse should be replaced by the word coition, which is the term used in the Repertory. 'Burning when urinating' appears to be a particular symptom, but of which part? The symptom of burning when he urinates is not clear enough, where is the burning? Usually it is in the urethra, but here it may be assumed to be in the glans. YOU MUST NEVER ASSUME ANYTHING WHEN PRESCRIBING, SINCE THE WRONG LOCATION COULD CHANGE THE SYMPTOM PICTURE AND THE REMEDY. You must determine exactly where the burning is, and not be shy to examine the patient. You cannot expect the patient to know clinical terms or to be familiar with the degree of precision you require. The examination of the patient is an important part of case-taking, and if you automatically attempt to complete each symptom according to time, location, sensation and modality you will get much of the accuracy and precision you require. For the sake of this exercise, we will assume the burning is in the glans.

ACTIVITY 2 List the symptoms above, then go through Kent's Repertory to find different rubrics for each symptom.

What Language Do We Use?

Of course this could also be entitled 'Which rubrics do we use?'.

If we take the first symptom, 'He finds it difficult to tell people he likes them because he fears rejection', then we end up with several rubrics. Fear of rejection is obviously a very real symptom which colours his day-to-day behaviour. It is not a feeling of being forsaken or abandoned, which appears in the Repertory, but a fear or anxiety, *but* there is no 'fear of rejection' in the Repertory. What is rejection? What other language can be found which expresses this state? A *fear of being unloved or of being alone*. 'Fear of being alone' can be found in the Repertory, but to this patient the fear is not of the present but the future. He does not want to be hurt any more. He does not know how he can face the hurt. **Anxiety about the future** may be a better rubric.

For the symptom 'unhappiness regarding his girlfriend' we have already said that we can use the rubric **Sad**.

The patient has twice said that he fears his girlfriend will reject him. Does his need to find security and settle down become a symptom? The patient wants to be loved and cared for. What is unusual about this? It is natural to want to be part of human society, however that is conceived. This patient is anxious that he will not achieve this, and he is also worried that his fears will spill out and he will show his anger at the present situation or at the past. Anxiety is a better word than fear to describe this, and is already contained in the selection of the rubric **Anxiety about the future**.

There are two powerful motivating forces in the case. One is the suppression of the anger, which he recognizes. The other is a recognition that something happened to him 7 years ago from which he has never recovered. He does not say what, but he states that he was very distressed when this relationship ended. Is it possible that **Worse disappointed love** is an exciting cause behind the presenting symptoms and behind much of his emotional turmoil? We have two other rubrics here. One is **Suppressed anger**, but there is also **Sadness after anger**, which may describe this patient.

He also describes himself as jealous and has grief. Both of these can be found as rubrics in the Repertory. Jealousy is a symptom given by the patient which gives rise to such questions as, 'What does he mean by jealousy when the patient *admits* it?' How jealous is he?

PRACTICE POINT When you are taking the case, ask yourself how many underlines you would give it so you can evaluate its intensity at the time. A good strategy is to ask the patient for an example if this is not given.

What language can we use to describe the fact that he would like to go away and visit friends? Is this:

- A desire for company?
- A desire to escape?
- Restlessness?

The continuation 'but feels lost and can't get it together' tends to suggest restlessness, but this could be a matter of degree depending on the judgement of the practitioner.

We are told the penis symptoms are worse after intercourse and masturbation. Note that in the case-taking process these come long after the original presenting symptoms, which were given at the start. Why? What exactly is aggravated by these modalities? In other words what is the symptom? We are inclined to take them as modalities of the part, but there is a possibility that they are generalities. In this case there is a considerable amount of emotion that the patient associates with sexual relationships. There is a considerable amount of energy expressing inner conflict, and there are many feelings that have not been integrated. This patient is indeed 'worse after coition' on the general level. Masturbation can be found under Genitalia, Masturbation, Disposition. In using this rubric we should think twice because in Kent's day it had more serious connotations than it has nowadays, and yet it does describe the patient, so it is included in our prescribing symptoms.

The Hierarchy of Symptoms

Since there are no other symptoms, you must now organize the hierarchy.

ACTIVITY 3

List the symptoms above into hierarchical order.
There are no strange, rare and peculiar symptoms, but there is an exciting cause and a very highly marked mental and emotional.

Disappointed love	Would seem to be the main exciting cause.
Suppressed anger	Is the most highly marked mental and emotional symptom.
Anxiety about the future	Describes the overall character of this patient.
Fear of losing control	Stems from the last two symptoms.
Restlessness	Also stems from the overall situation, or the patient's reaction to it.
Worse coition	Is the highest general which stems from the above, and has a qualitative effect on the presenting symptoms.
Masturbation	Describes a malfunction of sexual desire (or ability to express this).

Genitalia	**Inflammation**	**Penis**	**Glans**
	Pain	Sore	
	Redness		
	Pain	Burning	Glans
			On urination

These are the presenting symptoms, which are put at the end in this case because they are not serious, and because they belong to a part.

Hopefully you should have found the construction of a hierarchy quite simple by now.

The Repertorization Process

Now it is time to find a best-fit remedy.

Disappointed love	ant. c, *aur*, calc. p, caust, cimic, coff, hell, **hyos**, **ign**, *kali. c*, *lach*, **nat. m**, nux m, nux v, **phos-ac**, sep, staph, tarent.
Suppressed anger	aur, cham, *ign*, **sep**, **staph**.

The last symptom cuts out remedies and does not cover remedies such as **Nux Vomica**, which we would expect here from our knowledge of Materia Medica. Recent additions to the Repertory such as those of Vithoulkas include Nux Vomica under this rubric.

Sadness after anger   nux v, sep.

This rubric is too small to be useful.

If we were to take **Fear of being alone**, **Desires company** and **Desires to escape**, we would end up with the following:

Fear of being alone	hyos, **kali. c**, *nux v*, *sep*, tarent.
Desires company	kali-p, caust, **hyos**, *ign*, **kali. c**, **nux v**, *sep*, tarent.
Desire to escape	caust, hell, **hyos**, ign, lach, *nux v*.

Although there are common threads developing through these rubrics, the fact there are no remedies from the rubric **Suppressed anger** running through all of them should make us suspicious that all is not well. Remember that there are over 2000 remedy pictures, which is a phenomenal variety to choose from.

<table>
<tr><td>**PRACTICE POINT**</td><td>It is most unlikely that we have discovered the 2001st remedy picture! It is more likely that we have not got to the core of the case. To the beginner this is always a useful guide with which to evaluate our work.</td></tr>
</table>

Suspicion also arises when we turn to **Restlessness**, because a different group of remedies emerge. Once again I have used only those remedies already appearing under the rubric **Disappointed love**, because the final choice of remedy, whatever we arrive at, must contain the exciting cause.

Restlessness   aur, *caust*, *kali-c*, *lach*, *nat. m*, *nux v*, *phos ac*, **staph**, **tarent**.

If we continue along this line we must now add in the generals. The picture becomes clearer and there is now a distinct dominance of only a few remedies.

Worse coition	**kali. c**, nat. m, *nux v*, phos ac, **sep**, *staph*, tarent.
Masturbation disposition to	hyos, **lach**, nat. m, *nux v*, *ph-ac*, **staph**.

The local symptoms show a very limited choice, with few of our remedies appearing under the rubrics of the parts.

Genitalia inflammation, glans	*aur*, caust, lach, *nat. m*, nux v, phos ac, sep.
Genitalia pain sore	has no remedy
Genitalia restless	nat. m.
Genitalia burning glans	nat. m, phos. ac.

Selecting the Remedy

If we had followed this route of repertorization, we would have the remedies and values as in columns one and two below. Columns 2 and 4 contain the particular symptoms too.

	(1)	(2)	(3)	(4)
Causticum	5/5	6/6	5/3	6/4
Kali carbonicum	13/5		8/4	
Lachesis	8/4	9/5	9/4	10/5
Natrum Muriaticum	7/4	10/6	9/5	12/7
Nux vomica	13/8	15/11	9/5	11/7
Phosphoric acid	9/4	11/6	11/5	13/7
Sepia	10/6	11/7	5/3	6/4
Staphisagria	12/5		16/7	17/8
Tarantula	7/5		6/4	

The first figure is the number of points and the second is the number of rubrics under which the remedy appears. Hence 7/5 = 7 points and 5 rubrics.

As can be imagined with this volume of anger and unexpressed emotion, **Nux vomica** and **Staphisagria** are the prominent remedies; only **Kali carbonicum** is comparable. However, when the particulars are represented only **Nux vomica** holds its position, whereas **Phosphoricum acidum** and **Natrum muriaticum** are raised in value to become significant. **Nux vomica** now appears as a predominant remedy and by all standards is the one that should be chosen – by all standards, that is, except the Materia Medica.

Staphisagria and Nux vomica are very similar remedies, but it is Staphisagria that has the greatest degree of sexuality and effects from the suppression of sexuality, and this is the reason that I should select Staphisagria as the indicated remedy. How can this be justified? It does not come out well in the repertorization process. Anything could be argued with a Repertory. You could also choose Natrum muriaticum or Phosphoricum acidum.

Natrum muriaticum is a serious contender since it covers the exciting cause and the particular symptoms which are the presenting symptoms, but Natrum muriaticum does not have the anger of Staphisagria and Nux vomica. Phosphoricum acidum has the desire and sexuality of Staphisagria, but does not have the anger so highly marked.

Staphisagria is the only remedy for suppressed anger among these five and, as we agreed at the start, this is certainly the second most important symptom, if not the most important. Staphisagria is found under Genitalia inflammation, but not specifically under Glans. However, when the cause is removed the parts will be cured and, in this case, the parts can be ignored as secondary, so the exciting cause can be treated.

Now look at the repertorization below, in which I have changed three of the rubrics: **Fear of being alone**, **Desires company**, **Desires escape** for **Anxiety of the future** and **Fear of losing self-control**. The outcome is now very different:

Disappointed love	ant. c, *aur*, calc. p, caust, cimic, coff, hell, **hyos**, **ign**, *kali. c*, *lach*, **nat. m**, nux m, nux v, **phos. ac**, sep, staph, tarent.
Suppressed anger	aur, cham, *ign*, sep, staph.
Anxiety re future	ant. c, aur, *caust*, kali. c, *lach*, nat. m, *nux v*, phos. ac, *staph*, tarent.
Fear of losing self-control	*staph.*
Restlessness	aur, *caust*, *kali. c*, *lach*, *nat. m*, *nux v*, *phos ac*, **staph**, **tarent**
Worse coition	**kali c**, **nat. m**, *nux v*, *phos. ac*, **sep**, *staph*, tarent.
Masturbation	hyos, **lach**, nat. m, *nux v*, *phos. ac*, **staph**.
Genitalia inflammation	nat. m, nux v, sep, staph.

What a difference the language makes. The case is so much simpler. Staphisagria comes clear through all the rubrics as does no other remedy. The values as shown in columns 3 and 4 also show that it is far ahead of any other remedy.

In Summary

In taking the case we must seek clear precise symptoms and choose the rubrics carefully. The purpose of this lesson is to show you the importance of the right choice of language and prescribing symptoms. You could easily have ended up with a different choice of remedy by putting emphasis on different symptoms, or by repertorizing mechanically without combining a knowledge of the Materia Medica.

ACTIVITY 4 Rearrange the symptoms once again, or change the rubrics used to show you how other remedies can emerge.

ACTIVITY 5 Work through the following cases and see how many remedies you can get from the different use of language and prescribing symptoms.

1) Male, 3 years old.

A history of colds every 6 weeks, goes to the chest where he has wheezing respiration between 10.30 p.m. and 12.30 a.m. Since building work started on the flats opposite he has been worse. Since Christmas he has had regular coughing fits at 3 a.m. If he eats after 7 p.m. he vomits as soon as he lies down to sleep (which is around 8 p.m.) He prefers sweets, apples, carrots and cucumber. He drinks a lot. Expectoration is green and sometimes lumpy. He needs a lot of attention from Mum and he is preoccupied all the time. He is shy, and is ill if he goes to a party with strangers. He is stubborn and naughty – he hits people and always wants the last word. Possessive over toys and fights a lot. When not at playschool Mum often finds him playing quietly by himself. His sleep is restless and he often talks in his sleep. He prefers to sleep flat on his back. He chews his tongue in sleep. Fear of the dark. Vomits mucus. Cough is spasmodic. He has a history of frequent antibiotics since he was a baby; has been taking daily salbutamol for 1 year. Last month he was hospitalized for asthma attacks and was then given Theophylline. When ill his voice goes first, and he sneezes and brings up clear mucus that goes green and thick. When ill he is off food, is clingy and has a spasmodic cough.

2) Female, 28 years.

She has throbbing pain in the throat at the time of menstruation. The tonsils are so swollen they almost touch. They are agony to touch and worse for swallowing. When she coughs there is a pain between the shoulder blades. She has a history of athlete's foot, warts on the fingers that grow and drop off and grow again. The eyelids are dry and itchy, and she picks the scales off. There is a pain in the cervix that pulls down. The pain extends upwards from the cervix to the navel as if pulled by a string, before menstruation. Before menses there is also a throbbing pain in the right breast, and breast lumps grow in size. She could not care less about her husband and children before the menses. Now she is averse to salt. She has a fixation about cleanliness.

3) Female, 16 years.

The eczema, which is dry scaly eruptions, itches before bed. She is a fastidious person who loves chocolates, lemons and hot food. She sleeps with the light on because she is afraid of the dark. The patient is worse before menses and in wet weather.

4) Female, 34 years.

The toilet is an unpleasant experience. The bowels are loose and move several times in the day. There is tenesmus and the stool sticks to the rectum. The bowels never feel empty. She is tired in the afternoon and often falls asleep. Sadness before menses; the feet and ankles are swollen in the heat or before menses. Eyes are puffy in the morning; in the evening there are neuralgic pains, worse when she lies down. There is no sexual desire – feels irritated rather than turned on. She feels put upon – there is no climax or enjoyment in intercourse. She resents sexual contacts and hence has no children.

5) Female, 19 years.

A cyst in the right lower eyelid throbs when tired, or in the heat of summer. There is a hot pain in the inguinal area which appeared after a coil was put in for contraception. It has returned with every period since. Coil is now displaced and she is waiting to have it removed. A year ago she had an injury to her right wrist. Since then there is an aching pain at the base of the thumb, which is worse when she is tired. The abdomen is bloated before menses. She is lethargic in the heat but also suffers from cold. She prefers fresh air. She is worse for a change in the weather and is worse at the beginning of winter. She has a fear of heights and crowds. Lacks confidence, is weepy and depressed. With boyfriends she is fussy and finds it easier to communicate with women. She sleeps on her abdomen. Sleep is restless, circulation is poor. Parts quickly numb.

LESSON FOURTEEN

Case Analysis

Headings: Introduction
Nine Questions to Guide Case-Taking and Analysis
Case Example
Three Cases to Analyse Yourself

Aim: In this lesson you will be introduced to questions that will enable you to apply the homoeopathic philosophy to a patient's case.

Objectives: To recognize whether a case is acute, chronic or pseudochronic;
To identify an exciting or maintaining cause;
To be able to pick out the weak parts of the body;
To identify modalities.

Introduction

Finding a remedy involves a great deal more than just repertorization. It involves putting our philosophy to work to find out what needs to be cured, or how the vital force is disturbed. When we have analysed the case, we will know:

- *Which remedy to use.* In case analysis we recognize that it is possible that treatment other than a remedy is necessary. This involves an understanding of what it is that needs to be cured (para 71).
- *Which potency to use.* Potency selection requires a thorough understanding of the disease process in each individual case. The disease process is more advanced study.
- *How the patient will react to the remedy.* If we are to provide sufficient care of the patient, we must have some expectation of the action of the remedy. This last part is more advanced than I wish to cover here.

To me, case analysis starts while taking the case. Kent and others would disagree with this, saying the practitioner should not think of a remedy until all the information is collected. Although I agree with this emphatically, since to do so is to colour the data, to me taking the case is an active process and not as passive as Kent implies. It is not sufficient for a practitioner to act as a receptor: the practitioner is a question mark exploring a new field, tasting, testing and querying. Weighing the quality of the data involves assessment. The burning question in our minds is, What disturbed the vital force? This is very quickly followed by, Why can't the vital force correct the balance? The skills of case-taking fall into two categories.

- The practitioner needs interview and observation skills in order to obtain the information in its most accurate, precise and pristine form, uncontaminated. Case-taking is a skill that needs thorough training.
- The practitioner needs a thorough knowledge of homoeopathic philosophy, and the experience to apply this to the data.

The second may mean tracking down the exact point of origin of the disturbance, the exciting cause. It may involve a qualitative assessment of modalities, or of maintaining causes. When is an allergy an idiosyncrasy? When does a cold cease to be an acute and become the manifestation of a miasm? When is it necessary to make such distinctions during case-taking?

Nine Questions to Guide Case-Taking and Analysis

Before case-taking is complete we must have data to answer the following questions. There is no point in keeping your fingers crossed that you will have enough data. You must know enough philosophy to know you have the data needed to make sense of finding the remedy.

1) Is this an acute, chronic or pseudochronic case,
i.e. at what level are we treating?
2) What is the vitality of the vital force?
3) What disturbed the vital force or continues to disturb it,
i.e. the exciting cause, maintaining cause or miasm?
4) What changed after the disturbance,
i.e. how did the vital force respond to the disturbance?
5) To what is the vital force sensitive,
i.e. causation, predispositions?
6) When did the vital force produce symptoms,
i.e. exciting causes or modalities?
7) Where is the vital force manifest,
i.e. the location, which are the weak organs or predisposition?
8) What is unique and what is individual about this patient?
9) What stage has the disease process reached?

1) Acute, Chronic or Pseudochronic?

Each of these types of disease behaves in a different way and requires a different approach, so it is necessary to determine quickly which is being dealt with as the data required differ slightly.

Pseudochronic If the case is pseudochronic we will be more concerned with establishing the maintaining cause and correcting habit and environmental factors, such as diet, drugs, etc., which give rise to the condition. Such a case may not require medical treatment.

Acute In the acute disease there is usually a clear exciting cause plus a group of resulting symptoms, so the procedure we have already established will be simple, i.e. select the prescribing symptoms, form a hierarchy and repertorize the case.

While this may be sufficient, consideration of the long-term health of the patient requires that we recognize the predisposition, the underlying weakness that predisposes the patient to the acute. This may require deeper, more chronic treatment to strengthen the patient.

The acute illness is also linked to the vitality of the patient. The greater the vitality the less likely the patient is to be susceptible to the exciting cause, but the greater the vitality then the more sudden and violent the acute disease, because the reactions of the vital force are strong.

Chronic The treatment of the chronic illness needs a great deal more knowledge of philosophy than we have discussed up to this point. The analysis of such a case is nevertheless contained in the other questions. Put simply, we must identify the factors to which the vital force reacts, and the characteristic way in which it reacts. Consideration of vitality and how far the disease process has progressed will affect the treatment, as will events in the history of the patient's symptom picture. Treatment of the chronic disease is the treatment of the total symptom picture.

ACTIVITY 1   List the factors you need to know to determine whether a case is acute, chronic or pseudochronic.

Acute

Chronic

Pseudochronic

---

2) Vitality

This is a very important consideration of case analysis. Remember that disease affects the vital force depending on its vitality, predisposition and exposure to the exciting cause. So, when vitality is lowered the patient is more likely to become ill.

Vitality may be lowered by a number of maintaining causes, including lack of sleep, overwork and poor diet. Such a patient may be seen to respond to a particular exciting cause, and we may be tempted to emphasize this in our prescription, but a thorough analysis of the case could reveal the role of the maintaining causes which need attention to prevent further illness. Although the doctor would agree with this concept of vitality related to the disease, he would have difficulty with the following.

The homoeopath recognizes that the acute illness may arise out of the chronic disease when the vitality is sufficiently high for the vital force to attempt to throw off the chronic illness. The chronic illness suppresses the ability of the vital force to restore harmony. The disturbance that caused this has never been resolved. The vital force with more energy tries to complete the process by throwing out symptoms in an acute crisis. Since homoeopathic treatment facilitates this process, there is often an acute illness after treatment.

Such knowledge may affect our choice of potency. Treatment and potencies used should stimulate the vital force to act, but at a level within its capabilities – or vitality; it is important to assess this level during case analysis, or to ensure that the data on which to form an opinion are made available during case-taking.

3) What Has Disturbed the Vital Force?

This could be the most important information obtained during case-taking, as it may point to the exciting or maintaining cause, or to the point of change – that point at which the vital force was put off balance. It enables us to identify the morbific factor which was so great, or to which the vital force was so susceptible, that harmony could not be recovered. This is the point at which the symptom picture began.

On looking at the historical development of the symptom picture it may be obvious that this changed in response to specific causes. Case analysis should separate out the different stages of the disease process. Since the soil of the patient determines each subsequent reaction, there is a relationship between each development stage of the total symptom picture. Each stage will be relevant to the patient's current problems, but the most recent symptoms and the most recent point of change are the most important.

4) What Changed After the Disturbance?

Many remedies can be identified from the causation, but generally the choice is too broad, so we also need the pattern of changes produced (symptoms) to identify the remedy. Which symptoms are now most dominant, or how have they changed?

5) To What is the Vital Force Sensitive?

This is not necessarily the same as Question 3. We may refer to the underlying predispositions, the vital force's susceptibility, or we may refer to modalities that aggravate or ameliorate the symptoms.

115

ACTIVITY 2   List ten causative factors. The General section of Kent's Repertory may help you.

6) When is the Vital Force Sensitive?

Here we are referring to the time modalities, or yet again to predisposition. When did you become ill – in puberty? Puberty is a time and it is a process which drastically changes the rhythms and nature of the body. Is it therefore a modality or a causation, or the manifestation of a deeper weakness or predisposition? The answer may greatly change the way we look at the case.

ACTIVITY 3   Are you aware of any point at which your own health changed?
If not, perhaps that of a relative?

7) Where is the Vital Force Sensitive?

Each individual has characteristic weak parts which are affected by disease. Each remedy also has a symptom picture which contains characteristic patterns in each organ, so identification of these in the patient may help to match the remedy. For example, Pulsatilla and Silicea have throat problems that move into the ears, whereas with Sulphuricum it is the eyes that are next affected, but with Phosphoricum and Bryonia it is the chest.

The parts affected may also tell us much about the patient's vitality, e.g. when the disease manifests in the ears of the patient taking Silicea or Pulsatilla, we know there is less vitality than if it stopped at the throat symptoms. We will therefore alter our potency accordingly.

ACTIVITY 4   List as many things as possible to which you are sensitive.

8) Individuality

It is the primary goal of case-taking to find the nature of the patient and the amount of deviation from the norm, and to sum this up as the total symptom picture for which you must find a similimum. The question involves the synthesis of the whole case. What are the likes and dislikes? What is the temperament? It also asks what is it that stands out in this case, that which distinguishes it? This is more than simply a search for the strange, rare and peculiar symptoms.

ACTIVITY 5   Name other processes that change the rhythm and nature of the body.
When are you most likely to be ill?

9) The Disease Process

In the chronic case this is perhaps the most important question. It will tell us how the vital force has accommodated the disease and how volatile the balance is. It will also tell us the vitality available to correct the process and, along with the patient's history, it will tell us the route we have to trace to re-establish health, which, as Hahnemann said, 'is nothing but freedom from symptoms'. Sound knowledge of the Law of Cure will help here.

ACTIVITY 6   Go through as many of your family as possible and list those organs or anatomical processes that are affected when they are ill. Is there a pattern within the family?

In case analysis we have entered the realms of the art of homoeopathy, which can only be learned through practical application of the skills. So let us study a case.

ACTIVITY 7   As you read through the raw data below, pick out the prescribing symptoms.

Case Example

I have chosen the case of a dog because this immediately deprives us of much of the attitudes and prejudices with which we view our fellows. So we must work on the data. Such cases also involve our observation and deductive powers to the limit; children's cases can be similar.

Raw Data

A dog, 2½ years old, female bull terrier.

She has a great deal of hair loss from raw skin; it is almost all over but is worse around the genital area and in the 'armpits' and groin. As a pup she only had one patch, on her tail. This problem is common in bull terriers and is often aggravated by chalking the skin (coat) for shows.

She has been treated unsuccessfully with various steroids, cortisone and prednisolone had no effect, and have not controlled the situation that worsened 6 or 7 months ago.

'Heat' (a show of blood at ovulation) was absent at the last opportunity. She has had only two heats – in both she had milk in her breasts although not pregnant. The second developed into a false pregnancy when movement was visible in the abdomen. On the day of 'delivery' she was very anxious and discharged a green mucus-like fluid. When her owner touched her tummy it came out like a fountain.

She was vaccinated at 12 weeks and 16 months ago showed her second heat. The vaccination was for parvovirus and distemper.

She is very sensitive to heat and turns red when she sunbathes! (Even with 6 inches of snow outside, there is no heating on in the house as she goes much redder and goes crazy with itching). The patch on her tail started when she was 6 months old, which was also when the owner acquired another dog. This dog is jealous of the new one and bullies it, pushing it out of the way. Our patient is described as 'the boss'. She is not aggressive but very affectionate, and demands a great deal of attention. If she does not get this she is capable of stealing things and taking these to her basket, where she does not chew them but sits waiting for them to be collected. As she sits cuddling the dog, the daughter of the family describes her as 'wanting to be human' – indeed she sits on the daughter's knee most unlike a dog and more like a human baby.

She likes to please. If she is going to be sick, she waits for a bowl to be sick into! If she wets inside she is remorseful and goes about all day with her ears back.

She desires sweets, and is averse only to raw onions and such slimy foods as tongue. The mouth has a fishy smell.

She has a history of conjunctivitis and kennel cough. The conjunctivitis produced a pink discharge, but once again I was told that it is normal with this breed to have watery eyes in the morning. The kennel cough over 1 year ago was treated with antibiotics, but went on for 10 days as a dry cough with white phlegm. There is also a tendency for the right ear to be overwaxy.

Note: This is a useful place to point out that it is illegal to treat animals in the United Kingdom if you are not a registered veterinarian. This animal is treated with the permission of her vet.

The Prescribing Symptoms

It is not difficult to find the prescribing symptoms but in this case a lot of skill is needed to put them into a hierarchy. Also I have chosen this case because there is a chronology to the symptoms, and there are distinct exciting causes.

Presenting Symptoms

The presenting symptoms indicate one level of the disease:

Section	Rubric	T.L.S.M.	More detail T.L.S.M/Remarks
Skin	Red Raw Itching	Especially orifices Scratches until skin bleeds or red weals form	worse heat worse sun
Head(?)	Hair loss		Especially groin and armpits (?).
Generalities			Started on tail when she was a
117			puppy.

The last is the most important symptom since it goes back to the point of change. Is it the point of change, or the first appearance of a hereditary trait for which this breed is famed? How was the weakness activated? At present, we do not know.

Strange, Rare and Peculiar Symptoms

She has only had two heats.
She had milk in her breasts although not pregnant.
The false pregnancy with visible movement in the abdomen.
Green mucus-like fluid came out like a fountain.
She waits for a bowl to be sick into.

I have not put these symptoms into the language of the Repertory as I did with the presenting symptoms. To do so is already to decide on an interpretation, and I need to be careful here because this is a dog and I am using a Repertory of human symptoms.

ACTIVITY 8   List the different rubrics that might apply to the above strange, rare and peculiar symptoms.

Mental and Emotional Symptoms

We cannot speak to the dog so here we must go on our observations. There are some clear symptoms:

She is jealous, domineering of the other dog, affectionate to humans. She wants to please and is remorseful.

ACTIVITY 9   How would you interpret the symptom 'if she does not get attention she steals things, takes them to her basket, does not chew them but waits for them to be collected'?

General Symptoms

She desires sweets and is averse to raw onions and such slimy foods as tongue. There is not much to go on here.

ACTIVITY 10   Worse for heat is a very strong intensity.
Is this a general symptom or a modality of the part?

Particular symptoms

The mouth has a fishy smell. This is definite enough, but is it useful? The other skin symptoms belong under the presenting symptoms.

The Hierarchy of Symptoms

The next stage is to put the symptoms into a hierarchy.
   This is an interesting case with several strange, rare and peculiar symptoms, but there is a problem of language because she is a dog. How clearly can we interpret the patient's symptoms?
   The presenting symptoms have clear modalities. Can we treat these acutely?
   We must go back to the beginning and ask, what is it that needs to be cured in this patient? To what is the vital force reacting? What facts do we have?

She has had this problem since she was a pup.
This problem is endemic in the breed.

Both of these symptoms point to inherited chronic disease. Is there an exciting cause that might have caused such a deep disturbance so early on? i.e. was this level of disease inherited or did some factor bring out the underlying predisposition? Whatever the exciting cause, there must still be a predisposition to bring out and this is on the chronic level.

There is a chronology here. The problem got worse 6–7 months ago. Why? How did it get worse? i.e. how did the symptom picture differ, if at all? We are looking to see if the pattern progressed to deeper levels, or if it changed and took a different direction. Are there other points in time when the symptom picture changed? Look at the timescale:

Age	Change in symptoms	Event occurring
6 months	Disease appeared	New dog arrived
9 months	Milk in the breasts	First heat
15 months	False pregnancy	Second heat
21 months		No heat
2 years	Skin worse	
2½ years		No heat

The chronology shows up a pattern that was not obvious in the raw data. There is a disturbance in the reproductive system: the first heat brought the first strange, rare and peculiar symptom – milk in the breasts.

The second heat brought another strange, rare and peculiar symptom – false pregnancy. Then we have two heats missing. After the first of these there was a further degeneration in the skin. We can now see that the case is definitely on the chronic level, and probably miasmic, because of the continuing deterioration. Now we have answered our first question and commented on the second question, the vitality is continuing to degenerate. Now we must look more carefully at what disturbed the vital force.

Worse menstruation is the first factor we come across that disturbs the vital force. This ties in with our two strange, rare and peculiar symptoms, milk in the breasts during heat, and false pregnancy with movement in the abdomen and discharge of green fluid. It took some detective work to realize that the disease first appeared after a new pup had been acquired, of which the patient was very jealous. Is there other evidence to support this? Going back to the raw data we find that she is still jealous of the other dog and bullies it, pushing it out of the way despite the fact that she is described as not aggressive but affectionate.

We are looking at questions five and six. To what is the vital force sensitive, and when did the vital force produce symptoms? Let us look more clearly at the mental and emotional symptoms to help us here.

The dog is very sensitive as to how others will receive it or reject it. Look at these symptoms:

Very clean – waits for a bowl to be sick in;
Attention seeker – takes things to her bed and waits for the owner to collect;
Remorse if wets inside – goes around all day with her ears back.

Even if the owners have exaggerated, they are citing facts: her ears are back, she waits to be sick, she does not chew goodies but waits for them to be collected. We must then decide what language to use to describe this behaviour. What language would you use? Turn to your Repertory!

Demanding and attention-seeking are words we would commonly use today, but these are not to be found in the Repertory. **Affectionate** can be found there. **Remorse** can also be found there. Affectionate is backed by the daughter of the family, who treats her like a baby and states that she wants to be human.

Remorse is a very strong feeling. Can it be justified here? With animals it is more difficult to use Vithoulkas's system of underlining, but it is still necessary to weigh up the value of the symptom. The description of the dog going about all day with its ears back adds much significance to the symptom.

Question eight is answered by the fact that this dog does have a personality – it is jealous, affectionate, egocentric (bossy but not aggressive), wants to please, demands attention, it likes sweets but not onions or tongue. We have a language problem when we go to the Repertory. In order to find 'hair loss' we must look up in the Repertory

119

under 'Head', as it was written with humans in mind and they usually have hair only on the head. Similarly, the Repertory does not contain a rubric for 'worse ovulation', as this is usually an invisible process. Can we select 'worse menses' as the general rubric which shows a disturbance of the hormone cycle? Not really, as women often show a marked difference between these two points in the cycle. The show of blood in the dog is not menstruation. Are the hormones the same? This requires further investigation. However, we do have the two strange, rare and peculiar symptoms as part of our symptom picture, and they do answer question four, how has the vital force changed?

Now we have a better understanding of the case as to what changed, how it changed, and when it changed. To some degree we have even answered question nine, as to how the disease has progressed. Our hierarchy could now take on a different form:

Exciting cause	Jealous	anan, *apis*, calc. p, *calc. s*, camph, *cench*, coff, gal.ac, **hyos**, ign, **lach**, *nux v*, op, ph-ac, *puls*, raph, staph, stram.
S, R & P	Milk in non-pregnant	**puls**
	Movement in the abdomen	*calc. p*, coff, ign, op, *puls*, stram, sulph, **thuj**.
M/E	Affectionate	coff, *ign, nux v, puls*,
	Remorse	coff, *hyos, ign*, lach, nux v, *puls*, stram, sulph.
General	Amenorrhoea	*apis*, calc. s, *hyos, ign, lach, nux v*, ph-ac, **puls**, *staph*, stram, **sulph**.
	Worse becoming heated	calc. s, *camph*, coff, ign, nux v, *op*, **puls**, staph, *thuj*.

Analysis

Following my normal practice, I did not eliminate remedies at each successive stage of repertorization. All remedies hereafter are chosen from those appearing under the exciting cause, but I have also added **Sulphuricum** and **Thuja**. Had I chosen only the presenting symptoms, **Sulphuricum** would have come forward as the most obvious remedy, as there are two marked keynotes of **Sulphuricum**, namely redness around the orifices and the remarkable aggravation with heat. There is also another common symptom of **Sulphuricum**, the red weals after scratching. Had I not gone into such depth and treated the case acutely, then **Sulphuricum** would have been the most likely remedy to fit the symptom picture.

I have kept an interest in **Thuja** because it would have been the most likely remedy if I had been interested in the most strange, rare and peculiar symptoms of the false pregnancy with movement in the abdomen and the green fountain.

In looking at the total symptom picture and analysing the case thoroughly, there is only one remedy, **Pulsatilla**, which appears in all the rubrics. **Ignatia** appears in all but one, and **Coffea** and **Nux vomica** appear in all but two. **Sulphuricum** and **Thuja** are simply not prominent. The score is as follows:

Pulsatilla	17 points from 7 rubrics
Ignatia	9 points from 6 rubrics
Coffea	5 points from 5 rubrics
Nux vomica	8 points from 5 rubrics
Sulphur	5 points from 3 rubrics
Thuja	5 points from 2 rubrics

Pulsatilla is undoubtedly the leading choice when the case is judged on a points system. The Materia Medica tells us that **Pulsatilla** causes a need for a lot of affection and jealousy when this is threatened. Such a patient dominates social interaction with their needs for attention and approval, but will be acquiescent in behaviour so as not to alienate the source of attention. Does this agree with the information given in the raw data? Yes, I think so.

So, **Pulsatilla** was given. If it had been a human patient the remedy would have been used in a high potency, as indicated by the reactivity and the intensity of the symptoms and the fact that the disorder was still only on the level of organ function and not pathological change in structure, but with animals and children we use lower potencies because they are more sensitive.

ACTIVITY 11   Repertorize this case again, putting the emphasis on different symptoms, for example, the presenting symptoms or the strange, rare and peculiar symptoms.

ACTIVITY 12   Repertorize the case again using different language for the symptoms selected. For example, you could use 'desires company' instead of 'affectionate' or 'anxiety of conscience' instead of 'remorse'.

Three Cases to Analyse Yourself

Case 1

Male, 27 years.

Presenting symptoms: Thinning hair since two perms 9 months ago.
Current depression since 2 years.

History: Caesarean birth.
Breastfed.
Very naughty at secondary school!
History of colds since a toddler – at least every winter affected the chest and throat, green phlegm.

Chest: Sensation of a lump on the centre of sternum when he eats, first started when he started to jog 2 years ago.

Skin: Wart under left elbow, eczema on the back and front of hands in winter, worse when he was working in a wood factory 4–5 years ago. It was chipwood and he was exposed to a lot of resin, mainly smell. Skin is dry and scaly; there are no sensations.

Stomach: He has a preference for meat, salt, sweets, spicy foods. He is averse to orange peel in cakes, fatty meat and skin. He is worse only if he eats too much; if he eats late at night stomach is dodgy – very full as if there was a lump there. He has only had colic once a few years ago. He has a history of taking marijuana 6 years ago.

Bowel: Regular daily, sometimes twice. Pain on passing stool as if the anus were going to burst. Flatus smells of rotten eggs and is worse when he is nervous.

Mouth: Cracked and flabby tongue.

Head: Pain very rare – once he had three headaches in 1 week, across the forehead and throbbing in nature. He was then very nauseous and vomited. He also gets nausea if he goes out jogging just after he has eaten. More commonly he has a heaviness in the stomach when he does this.

Urine: Bright yellow with acrid smell.

Sweat: Profuse when he walks vigorously or jogs, as if he is nervous or in a crowded place. He sweats mainly on the axilla, crotch and back. Sweat smells sour.

Sleep: Five hours each night then catnaps between 1 and 2 hours. He feels he never has enough. He is dopey on rising and takes half an hour to wake up if at work, 1 hour if at home. He says he is worse after sleep. He is irritable when tired. He dreams of being a hero and indulges in his dream escapades directing his activities in dreams. The sleep position is fetal, on the right side. He does not feel comfortable on the left side.

Weather: In the heat he is tired and sweats a lot. Hands are worse in the cold – they are like blocks of ice. His eyes are affected by the sun. He likes the seaside because he fishes.

Family history: Maternal grandmother died of a broken heart.
His sister had TB in one lung
Another sister suffers from bronchitis but she smokes.

Mind: He is irritable if someone does something stupid; he cannot reason with them. He tells them off. It is worse when he is tired. He cries at sentimental films. Anger if others insensitive – he just walks off.

Anxious meeting people for the first time, or new situations.

Shy about women and personal questions.

He cannot concentrate in noise.

He likes music and dance.

He is sad if something happens to his friends. He sits quietly and thinks of it.

He dislikes sympathy because exposure embarrasses him.

Very untidy. Stubborn – he thinks carefully before he makes a decision, so will not change it easily.

Insecure. Fears rats, mice, cockroaches and spiders.

He is of a happy disposition and finds it difficult to be serious. Emotional shock a couple of years ago (!). He will not discuss this, but says he has since felt resentment, anger and shame. He cried then and still does so now when he thinks about it, but it does not stop him from getting to sleep. He felt rejected. He does not tell people what is wrong with him.

ACTIVITY 13 Pick out the prescribing symptoms, put these into a hierarchy, then repertorize the case.

Additional questions for this case:
Label at least three maintaining causes. One of these needs to be confirmed – what question would you ask to clarify this?

Label two exciting causes and name which symptoms appeared after each of these. Which is the most important exciting cause?

Describe the character of this patient.

Case 2

Female, 55 years.
Presenting symptoms: General malaise started 5 years ago after an operation for cancer, extended hysterectomy. Antisocial and cannot be bothered to talk. Her father was killed 6 years ago and she has had health

problems ever since. Her husband died of cancer and she had to bring up the children on her own. She now feels it was all pointless. Before this her only problem was PMT; now she has backache and a boring pain in the kidney area. She gets very hot then cold in bed, and has very hot palms.

History: As a child she was very nervous.
As a teenager she was very lively and did not have colds.

Genitalia female: PMT developed after her husband died. Before that she had backache only before menses, but now has tension and irritability.

Chest: Asthma developed after her husband died. She could not walk without wheezing. It went suddenly when she moved house. High blood pressure developed 6 months after her father died.

Sleep: She describes herself as too tired to sleep. She is tired all the time, she wakes tired. She sleeps on her left side, she is too hot or cold in the night, and worse for covering.

General: She has put on weight since the death of her father.

Extremities: She has developed an aching pain in her knees over the last 6 months.

Ears: Over the last 6 months she has developed a high-pitched screaming in these.

Head: Pains develop during PMT, worse for alcohol or talking to someone she would rather not be talking to! The pain starts from tension in the neck area.

Stomach: She desires salt, sweets, vinegar, peppers and is averse to fat.

Skin: Dry and puffy around the ankles and wrists.

Mouth: Over the last 6 months she has developed mouth ulcers.

Sweat: Sour smelling, profuse under the arms, and after exertion.

Weather: No longer likes the heat (recent), prefers the rain and changing seasons. She likes the cold and the snow.

Mind: Concentration is so poor she fears driving.
Grief: Her sister died 5 months ago. She feels so guilty that she felt like dying. Weeps from music. Averse to company because she does not have the energy to put on an act that all is well when it is not.

Fear of being alone at night, of being ill, of not being able to work, as she is thus dependent on others.

Anxiety in case something happens to her children.

Additional questions for this case:
Visualize the patient clearly. What symptoms above best help you to describe her?

How many points of change are there in this case?

How do these demonstrate a change in the disease process through change of rhythm to pathological change?

At what point would you place the sensation stage of the disease?

Case 3

Female, 41 years.

Presenting symptoms: Pain from elbow down into hand, started on the right and now on the left.
Numbness on the arms worse gripping or exertion – she loses feeling in the arms.
This started 13 years ago after she very vigorously rubbed a floor. She can wake in the night with excruciating pain, it is better if she holds her arm straight up in the air.
The pain comes in the middle of the night, the numbness during the day.

Mind: She feels her memory is going fast since last year. It is like a fog. Once she could remember conversations she had had, not now.

Head: Hair falling at an alarming rate since 10 years ago. It is now thin, worse at the sides.

Extremities: The varicose veins on the outer side of the thighs prickle, especially on the right side.

Eyes: Vision has deteriorated in the last 2 years.

Abdomen: It feels tight and hates clothes around the waist.

Stomach: Good appetite unless depressed; says she eats for comfort. Desires cream cakes, tea, sweets and salt. Worse garlic, alcohol and tobacco.

Bowels: Can be loose. She has had piles since 1 year ago.

Urinary: Consumes 3 pints of fluid daily. Urinates frequently. Wakes to go to the toilet just after midnight. Pyelonephritis 14 years ago affected the right side and recurred for 8 years.

Genitalia female: Menses did not occur until 16 years old. Periods were irregular and there is a history of amenorrhoea. Breasts are tender for a few days before the period. Leucorrhoea between the periods – white sticky, and twice bloody recently.

Ears: History of earache when younger, worse right ear.

Mouth: Receding gums. White eruptions on tongue, red on the side of the mouth, better sticking out tongue.

Eyes: Bloodshot, dry – worse reading in the evening, sensation as if a wind blowing past them.
Lachrymation, worse in the wind.
Black spots float across the vision from left to right.

Skin: Eruptions throughout teens, more on each cheek.
Peduncular warts under both arms.
Warts on fingers of the right hand came on the same day (when 16 years old) that father's went.
Blood-filled vesicles right side of trunk.
Dry skin, scaly dry rash moves from right to left.

Extremities: Aching pain in the knees, worse for damp and exertion.
Knees crack and are stiff a lot.

Sweats: All the time if nervous. It smells aromatic, as if she has eaten spices. She may awake soaked but usually worse on her hands.

Sleep: She dreams of cakes and falling. Before stressful events she has nightmares. If she wakes in the night it is difficult to get off again because her mind is so active. She wakes with her jaw rigid and tense. She jerks before going off to sleep. She dribbles in sleep.

Weather: She finds thunderstorms exciting.
She dislikes stuffy heat.

History: She was a forceps delivery, breastfed. Tonsils and adenoids were removed when she was 5. Nightmares started after a car crash 18 years ago.
She had another crash 4 years ago.

Mind: Sad and depressed for years.
She weeps a lot – she has a sense of failure and always wanted to be liked and special. She pushes people to the limits to get them to reject her. She wants people to give their all to her. She says her own centre rests in others.
She feels empty and worthless, terrified of everyone. She says all was taken away from her and given to her sister.
When she left her home country she did not see anyone for 6 months.
She had therapy for 3 years.
She lacks confidence in groups or with authority.
She says she never faces fear or pain.
She is afraid of other's anger, or if they do not totally love her. (She does not open letters for 1 week sometimes).

She cries when frightened and wants to run away and hide in a little hole in the earth and go to sleep.

Anger boils over into temper but she says she is not assertive. She hates to be trampled on or to see others trampled on. She feels misery or hatred.

Moods alternate.
She loves being outside.

She fears to be alone as it is as if she did not exist. In the last few years she does not talk about her feelings, but shuts herself away and does not want to be comforted.

She hates new clothes because it exposes her and she has something to live up to then.

She is recently aware of a feeling of being smothered.

Additional questions:

From the evidence available, organize this patient's symptoms in chronological order.

Select three symptoms that most express her mental state. Have any changes occurred in these over time?

READINGS

Vithoulkas G *The science of homoeopathy*, Chs 13 & 14
Kent J T *Lectures on homoeopathic philosophy*, Chs 32 & 33

ADDITIONAL READING

Miller R J *Comparative value of symptoms in selection of the remedy.* Jain, New Delhi

APPENDIX I

Hints to Aid Study

There are two aspects of study that plague students of any age:

- A need to understand the subject matter;
- A need to recall the subject matter, i.e. memory.

Understanding Material

The crux of this is expressed in many examination questions which ask the student to explain in his or her own words.

When dealing with material, break it down into sizeable chunks and attempt to summarize in your own words, or to express in diagrammatic form or in a flow chart. The method you select may well depend on the subject matter. During this process of analysis you will be able to **separate out exactly which sentence, concept or group of words is giving you problems**, and you can then adopt various strategies for dealing with this. Usually it involves having the problem sentence defined in other words or, if a concept, in diagrammatic form; doing this yourself helps greatly, but a teacher or fellow student might help with examples to help you 'see the light'. This expression, 'see the light', tells us what is happening or needs to happen. You will understand if the concept is **explained in terms that touch your own field of experience**, i.e. in terms with which you can identify.

Knowledge is like increasing concentric circles of light with you at the centre (Fig. A1). Each part is connected. *If A lies in the dark part of the circle, it may not help you to know what A is because it lies totally outside your field of experience – the lighted circle – so we must build a pathway through B*, the less dark area. A properly designed curriculum will do this for you as it unfolds the subject matter in graduated steps; many activities in this text are designed to test each step as you go along. A tutor will identify your individual areas of isolation and give you special help to build bridges. However, if you are familiar with this process you can build your own bridges by first identifying the dark areas you need to know about. You may then be able to tackle individual words and concepts using a dictionary or the relevant pages of a textbook. Most modern textbooks present material more than once in different ways, e.g. diagrams and examples back up text, and you can use these side by side with difficult passages. If you still do not understand a concept it may be because some facts are taken for granted at this level, and you may have to go to a more basic textbook or a reference book, which should explain things so they can be understood at all levels. Teachers can also make it so much easier.

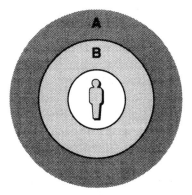

Fig. A1

Apart from missing stages, **the usual stumbling blocks are technical words and weighty grammar**. The subject you have chosen to study, homoeopathy, has special areas of difficulty here. There is *medical terminology* with which you should become familiar as soon as possible. It will be easier if you have already done a course in anatomy and physiology. Even so, you may find it useful to have access to a medical dictionary. A standard dictionary is also useful when studying homoeopathy, because some of the texts we use are over 100 years old and their authors often use words that would now be considered pedantic or obscure. Many of their medical terms are so old they are more often found in the standard dictionary than in the medical dictionary. Keep a notebook and write down unusual words you come across in homoeopathic books. If you cannot find a meaning for these, take them to your teacher or tutor, if you have one. Add them as questions at the end of your homework. If they arise during lectures and influence your understanding of a whole area of work, then of course you should bring this to the attention of the lecturer. Do not hesitate, because you may not be the only one who is lost and more shy classmates may be grateful.

In the days when these books were written there was a fashion to write **very long-winded sentences, which frequently obscures meaning**. As we study the *Organon* we will become especially aware of this. For example, paragraph 11 contains the following:

> 'When a person falls ill, it is only this spiritual, self-acting (automatic) vital force, everywhere present in his organism, that is primarily deranged by the dynamic influence upon it of a morbific agent inimical to life; – it is only the vital force, deranged to such an abnormal state, that can furnish the organism with its disagreeable sensations, and incline it to the irregular processes which we call disease; for, as a power invisible in itself, and only cognizable by its effects on the organism, its morbid derangement only makes itself known by the manifestation of disease in the sensations and functions of those parts of the organism exposed to the senses of the observer and physician, that is, by morbid symptoms, and in no other way can it make itself known.'

How does one make sense of this *one* sentence? First, we recognize that most of it is adding more explanation or detail to the central point, so we must **identify the central point** and separate it from its surroundings. We can only make sense of the rest if we see it as made up of adverbal or adjectival clauses, which further explain the verb or the noun, e.g. 'everywhere present in his organism' describes the vital force, a noun. Also, excess material is frequently in parenthesis, in brackets, or within commas, or split off from the main text by dashes. These play havoc with the understanding when they appear in the middle of the central theme, or when numerous of them are tagged on at the end of the central theme. Without a very good grasp of grammar this sentence is horrendous. For example, did you realize, without reading it four times like me, that he was saying four things:

1) When a person falls ill, it is only the vital force that is deranged;
2) It is only the vital force that can furnish the organism with its disagreeable sensations;
3) This vital force is invisible;
4) It only becomes manifest in the production of disease symptoms.

One way of coping with this sentence might be to underline the verbs, then rule out any phrase that does not have a verb or that cannot stand and make sense by itself, even with a verb. Thus:

> When a person <u>falls ill</u> it <u>is</u> only this spiritual, self acting (automatic) vital force, everywhere present in his organism, that <u>is</u> primarily <u>deranged</u> by the dynamic influence upon it of a morbific agent inimical to life; it <u>is</u> only the vital force, <u>deranged</u> to such an abnormal state, that <u>can furnish</u> the organism with its disagreeable sensations, and <u>incline</u> it to the irregular processes which we call disease; for, as a power invisible in itself, and only cognizable by its effects on the organism, its morbid derangement only <u>makes</u> itself <u>known</u> by the manifestation of disease in the sensations and functions of these parts of the organism <u>exposed</u> to the senses of the observer and physician, that <u>is</u>, by morbid symptoms, and in no other way can it <u>make</u> itself <u>known</u>.

Once you have the central theme with its subject, verb and object **go back over the full sentence** and **see how each clause you threw out changes the meaning of the central theme**, or **helps to explain it further**. Thus:

'When a person falls ill . . .'	He is talking about a special circumstance.
'spiritual, self-acting, (automatic) . . .'	These are all adjectives that further explain the nature of the vital force.
'everywhere present in his organism'	Again this explains a bit more about the vital force, that is is found everywhere in the organism.
'by the dynamic. . inimical to life'	This emphasizes *how* the vital force becomes deranged.

Thankfully, not all sentences are as gruesome as this, but this technique of breaking things down grammatically you should find useful to understand better what you read. Although at first you may have to write everything down, you will find before long that you can do it automatically in your head as you go along. A problem I often find with adult learners is disillusionment, because they think at their age they should know that fact or skill, so they are humiliated. You cannot cheat the learning process. Each stage must be gone through, first crawling and then walking. If you accept this and go for each stage you can accelerate the learning process, so usually adults learn faster.

Notice that as I go through *this* text, I am highlighting the main themes that I want you to grasp.When you are studying a text you may find it useful to **underline or highlight the main points**, what you think are the author's main points, and which points are most important to you as a student.

You can take this further **by adding concordant thoughts in the margin**, tracing the line of connection from one area or subject to another, e.g. from homoeopathy to anatomy. When you study you are thinking and linking new knowledge into boxes, or frames of reference, that you have already. Thus in exploring your theme you are widening your concentric circles of knowledge. If you do think actively and consciously you will accelerate the learning process. This is important in homoeopathy because we study humans, and such is the variety that we will go on studying as long as we practise. As homoeopaths we need to **see things from many different angles**. The number and the type of cases we can treat is limited by our field of experience. (Dorothy Shepherd used to read the *Sporting Life* regularly so she could talk to some of her patients!)

Memorizing Material

This is easier once the material is understood. It is also much easier if we know how the mind works. There are several characteristics that make recall easier. The most important is that *the mind works in patterns*, hence diagrams are easier for most of us to 'learn' than pages of words. This should affect *the organization of your notes*. The *shape* of these could aid memory. Some of the following points may help:

1)   Notes should be clear and concise; cut the waffle.
2)   Organize layout to help clarity, e.g. start new points on a new line, or put boxes around important information so it stands out. Use space well – once again, think in patterns.
3)   Use titles and subtitles and clearly differentiate these, e.g. put capitals in titles and underline; underline subtitles.
4)   Underline or highlight central themes, concepts or main points.
5)   Number points and subpoints.
6)   Explain where necessary and always give examples. This is necessary strategy for examinations.

7) Use diagrams wherever possible to summarize text. Again, this is essential strategy for examinations (Fig. A2).

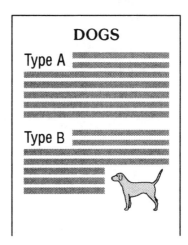

Fig. A2

While organizing the shape of your material do not forget its *content*.

Learning lists of facts is inefficient.

Organize material so that concepts are highlighted. **Learn the essence of the process that links the facts**, or **draw a flow chart**. Go over the text, sorting out what is important and why, just like you did when you were reading the textbooks. Again, **you are looking for patterns**.

FLOW CHART

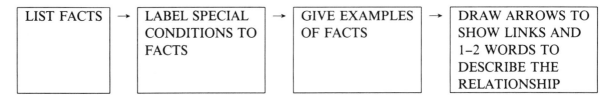

The second main characteristic of mind is that *it can only focus on one thing at a time*.

One side of this coin is attention, and the other is concentration. If we also remember that *the focus of the mind prefers to move continually*, then we either have a recipe for disaster or an idea for strategy. The mind remembers better if it is interested. Think of the mind of the child, who learns so much each day. The interested mind is mesmerized in one subject, but even though lost in concentration it keeps moving, problem-solving around one issue. The following points may help you apply this little bit of knowledge practically to your study:

1) Given a subject, cut out all diversions; *the more attention* you can give, *the greater the consciousness* you can achieve, and therefore the more likely you are to remember.

2) Take your subject and give the mind problems to solve; ask it questions – playing games with a child helps it to learn, maintains its attention. This is *active learning*. Anyone will learn better if they are involved *or take part*. These games can build up patterns and associations which further enhance the learning experience.

   How do you play games with yourself? It may be simply covering the page and writing down the main points that you have just read. You can pull out key words from the text then rebuild the text without consulting the original – this has the benefit of also concentrating on understanding.

3) In straight memory exercises we should recognize that *the mind can only concentrate for very short periods* – one minute or less – before it starts to wander, so **we must feed it little chunks**, a few sentences or a theme, and then **either take a break or change the subject**. With the mind it really is a case of a change being as good as a rest. We will get more out of the mind if we organize our study day

with regular breaks and a change of subject periodically. And of course we must take adequate exercise, fresh air and food to maintain a healthy environment for the body.

4)   Another useful hint to help you remember is that *the mind focuses on things that stop and make it hesitate, that do not fit neatly into its frames of reference*. We can use this in different ways to help us remember. **We can put familiar thoughts into different words or context.** We can make jokes or cartoons. We can surprise ourselves.

You will find that there are books available specifically on study skills and you may want to use one of these to take this matter further if you have not been involved in study for some time.

APPENDIX II

Guidelines on conducting a proving;

from the Society of Homoeopaths Research Group
Chairman: David Munnings

Concerning the supervisors of provings.

a. Quality of persons — supervisors should have completed a 3-year course with an *accredited* college and have commenced to practise, or supervisors should be members of the Society's Register.

b. Instructions

    (i) Provers should be identified by number and all sections of the case should be kept confidential.

    (ii) The identity of the prover should not be revealed to other provers.

    (iii) Supervisors should not discuss the proving with the prover or anyone likely to be known to the prover.

    (iv) The case should be taken in a logical schematic form and include appearance, modalities, family history and personal history – vaccinations, accidents, operations, etc.

    Schema: Mind, Vertigo, Head, Eyes, Nose, Face, Mouth, Teeth, Ears, Throat, Stomach, Abdomen, Rectum, Stool, Urinary, Male or Female Genitalia, Chest, Cough, Expectoration, Respiration, Back, Arms and Legs, Sleep, Chill, Fever, Perspiration, Skin, Generalities, Modalities, Sensations, Family History and Personal History.

    Objective tests should include blood pressure, temperature under left and right arm, urine samples and pulse rate.

    (v) Make sure the prover understands all instructions and note-taking. Explain the symptoms diagram. Impress on them the importance of detail.

    (vi) The prover should be seen once a fortnight and the schema gone through each time. This will go on till Week 6 then at the discretion of the supervisor.

    (vii) The prover is to have placebo for the first 2 weeks.

    (viii) After the first 2 weeks unsuitable provers will be eliminated from the trial. These will include people taking drugs of any kind except alcohol in moderation, herbal treatment, or persons who have pathological changes, are uncooperative or have hypersensitivity diseases.

    (ix) The proving should end when:

        a. the symptoms cease;

        b. if the symptoms continue too long or prove to be too severe, it may be desirable to find a suitable antidote, i.e. the higher potency;

        c. the prover, or relatives, get alarmed by the symptoms;

        d. any pathology appears – even a sore throat is a sign to stop;

        e. chronic symptoms are cured.

    (x) The prover should stop taking the remedy as soon as symptoms appear.

    (xi) The organizers should be contacted in ANY emergency.

    (xii) All information should be sent to the organizers at the end of the proving. The salient parts of this should be typed up in schematic form.

Dear Prover;

by Jeremy Sherr as appearing in the proving of Scorpion 1982. Taken from 'Guidelines to Provers'

Note-taking

When taking part in a proving the most important factor is accurate and full recording of all symptoms. Please do this in a new notebook (and not separate pages), marked with your prover's number. Since this will be presented to your supervisor on each visit you may find it useful to have two books which are alternated.

Begin by writing down all your current symptoms and a brief medical history. Record the marking on your pills and the amount to be taken daily.

When you commence the proving, note down carefully any symptoms that arise. This should be done as frequently as possible so that the facts will be fresh in your memory. Make a note even if nothing happens. Each day record the times of taking the remedy.

The following factors are important in noting symptoms: location, sensation, modalities, time and intensity.

Location	Try to be anatomically accurate. A drawing of precise location is very helpful. Note if the symptoms extends in any direction.
Sensation	Burning, sharp, dull, etc.
Modalities	What makes the condition better or worse, e.g. types of weather, sitting, standing, cold heat, movement, lying down, dark, pressure, etc. Find out.
Time	When do symptoms occur? When are they better or worse?
Intensity	Please underline any symptoms of strong intensity.

Next to any symptoms please note, if applicable, if you have had this symptom before, or if it is unusual for you or even highly unusual.

Also, note any long-standing symptoms of yours that have disappeared or grown worse.

Occasionally go over the schema (head, nose, eyes, etc.) to make sure you have missed nothing.

Mental and emotional symptoms are most important – please describe these accurately.

Give full descriptions of dreams if possible.

Reports from friends and relatives can be very enlightening. Please note if possible.

At the end of the proving, please note how you feel the proving affected you in general. Has your health improved, deteriorated, or remained the same? Give examples or reasons.

Please remember accurate symptoms make valuable proving!

On Taking the Remedy

The remedies should be taken regularly only until *definite* symptoms arise, after which time *no more* of the remedy should be taken; if in doubt at all stop taking the remedy. This does not mean the proving is over: symptoms should still be recorded until you are sure there are none left. Consult the supervisor.

Do *not* begin taking the remedy again once you have stopped.

During the proving avoid all antidoting factors such as coffee, camphor, peppermint, menthol and eucalyptus.

Keep your symptoms to yourself – do not compare notes with fellow provers until the experiment is over and the notes have been handed in. Your identity should be known only to the supervisor.

Finally, thank you for participating in this proving. There is no better way of learning and advancing homoeopathy. And, as J.T. Kent says in his *Lectures on Homoeopathic Philosophy*: 'A proving properly conducted will improve the health of anyone. It will help them turn things into order. It was Hahnemann's advice to young men to make provings'.

NB: Some provers will be given placebo. Even the supervisor will not know who has this. It is standard double-blind technique to ensure honest reporting of symptoms.

APPENDIX III

Some Model Answers to Activities

Lesson 4

| *ACTIVITY 9* | A hierarchy may be constructed as follows: |

1) *Introverted since the accident 16 months ago which she thinks she caused.*
This comes first since it contains the exciting cause, underlined.
Flies into a rage when the accident is mentioned.
This is the reaction to the accident, and is of such an intensity that could be a very good reason to put it first.
Hides behind mother when entering a room where a stranger is present.
This symptom expresses an inability to adapt to a social situation.
Sits sucking thumb.
I have put this next as it is an M/E symptom.

Chilly ⎫ Both these symptoms are generals. I have put them in this order
Fatigued ⎭ because fatigue is more common – it appears in many ailments.

Blond hair.
This is a physical characteristic with little prescribing importance except that it often indicates lax tissue type, but that does not mean that all Scandinavians are lax in tissue.

2) *Sweats on the face while eating.*
This is put first as the only S,R&P.
Weeps without cause.
This comes next as the only M/E.
Worse fasting ⎫ Both are general symptoms and an argument could be put
Worse before menses ⎭ forward to put either first. In case analysis we would select as more important the one that causes the greatest changes.
Worse cold food and drink.
This is also a general symptom but with more local causation, so I have put it after the other two.
Thirst for large quantities.
This is also a general, but one which implies choice. If you read the essays at the beginning of your repertory you might find a reason to put this higher up in the hierarchy.
Constipation with hard, dry stools.
Constipation is a general symptom showing the state of the metabolism, though in certain individuals it may tell us more about individual organs, such as the liver.
Backache worse lifting things, better rubbing and heat.
This is the presenting symptom but, although it has clear modalities, it is put at the end as a particular.

3) *Epistaxis when menses are absent.*
This is general and S,R&P, and so is put at the top of the list.
Black blood forms in long threads.
This is also S,R&P but is put second as it is only a particular.

Anger before lunch }
Anxiety prevents sleep } Both are M/E but anger is put first as more volatile.
Dissatisfied with job.
Although this is an M/E it is quite common or even justified in today's world. It must be more intense before it is placed higher up in the hierarchy.
Numbness on the right side.
This general symptom is highly individualized, occurring on the right side only. If highly marked we might even consider putting it in third place.

4) The order in this case depends very much from which angle it is looked at. I am not surprised to hear different versions from students. In practice there is less of a problem because the patient will put an emphasis on what is important in his/her case.
Nausea even with the smell of food.
This is a perversion of what should be a useful function, stimulating appetite.
Loathing of food.
This could join the first symptom for the same reasons.
Simultaneous vomiting and diarrhoea.
This is S,R&P.
These symptoms might be put first in an acute case but might be relegated to the particulars in a chronic case.
Sudden unaccountable fear.
This is a marked M/E.
Wakes 4 a.m. with anxiety.
This is an M/E with a clear modality.
Worse while alone.
This is an M/E.
Restlessness.
This is an M/E symptom too but a little too vague as it stands.
Desires alcohol, especially brandy.
This is a general symptom of appetite.
Abdominal pain, burning, better hot applications.
This is a clearly marked particular symptom with sensation and modality.
Urine scant and burning.
This is a particular symptom of little distinction.
Limbs cold.
This is also a particular symptom, but is put after the last because it is simply a change in rhythm, whereas the above burning is more destructive.
Colic.
This is simply the description of abdominal pain.
When you have learned to repertorize, go back to this case and repertorize it in different ways to see if your result changes.

5) *Shrieks before convulsions.*
This is S,R&P and M/E.
Thirstlessness.
This is a general, but S,R&P in a state of fever.
Dry heat and sweating alternate.
This is a peculiar individuality of the general symptom of fever.
Irritable when roused.
This M/E symptom shows how this patient is dealing with this situation. There is an argument to put this symptom before the last, as it is M/E.
High temperature }
Worse hot baths } These three symptoms clearly go together. The fever is a general. The other two are common in fever, and are
Better cold application } not worth noting except to differentiate remedies.
Stiffness of neck accompanies convulsions.
This is a particular symptom, but also relatively common in some kinds of convulsions. It is an important symptom, showing the seriousness of the physiological situation, i.e. the involvement of cerebrospinal fluid.

6) *Fear of men.*
    This is an unexpected symptom in a social animal such as a human. Thus it is given the place of a S,R&P and M/E symptom *unless* there is a sound reason such as sexual abuse.
    Fear of dogs.
    In comparison to the above this is simply an M/E symptom.
    Tearful.
    This M/E tells us about the personality of the patient.
    Cough dry and teasing, persistent.
    This is a particular symptom showing changes in the important respiratory system. Now we have a problem. Are we making an assumption that the three modalities belong to the cough, i.e. < breathing in, < in a warm room, < lying down? If this is so there is no problem, but they could be general modalities of the patient. In taking the case you must never leave this question open.
    Warts on the left hand.
    This particular is put last as having less effect on the patient's life than the cough.

7) *Cold exterior with internal heat.*
    This is not an easy symptom to diagnose, but once found it is S,R&P.
    Apathetic and indifferent.
    This is the only M/E symptom.
    Great desire for fresh air.
    This is an intense general symptom.
    All of the other symptoms are particulars and are therefore grouped according to their strangeness, to their seriousness or degree of contribution to the whole, or to their clarity – that they have clearly marked modalities. Hence:
    Tongue feels cold.
    This is a strange symptom.
    Bluish pallor around the mouth.
    This is distinctive and also hints at a change in the general state of the organism. Although it probably is a general state, we do not give it that status as the symptom stands.
    Puffy hands.
    This is similar to the above and is put next because it has slightly less information.
    Swollen parotid glands.
    This particular symptom is put next as part of the lymph system that drains the whole body.
    Itching and burning of the private parts.
    This is a more localized symptom than the last, even though it could be argued to cause more distress.
    Putrid flatulence.
    I have put this last as it is the product of an organ – the intestines.

8) There are only four non-particular symptoms in this case. Two of these, dislikes work and obesity, may be too 'common' and a result of today's culture and habits. They must be very highly marked to be of use. However, if we take the data as given we might end up with the following hierarchy:
    Music saddens and causes to weep.
    This is almost S,R&P.
    Peevish and whiny.
    This describes the temperament of the individual.
    Dislikes work.
    This is an M/E describing 'desires and appetite'.
    Obesity.
    This is a general symptom describing metabolism.
    Head feels numb and empty.
    I have put this first of the particulars since it is on the sensation level of disease and in this case very individual.
    Headache with pressing pains on the vertex.
    This particular goes next because it has the clearest modalities.

Burning pains in the abdomen.
Excoriation of flexures and sweating parts.
The last comes after 'abdomen' as the lesser organ. Neither has clearly marked modalities.
Running sores behind the ears.
Although describing a more specific area than the above two particulars, this is more vague and urgently requires detail, e.g. what is running out of the ear – colour, consistency, etc.?
Foul odour from breath.
This could also be described more accurately. I have put it last, as being least serious of the last three particulars.

9) The presence of hydrothorax, a serious organ disturbance, complicates this case. If acute it may require our most urgent attention but, if ongoing and chronic, may represent no more than pathology in an organ. I have taken it as the latter below and relegated it to the bottom.
Construct another hierarchy putting it at the top.
Flies into a rage on exposure to strong light.
This is an inexplicable S,R&P symptom, also on the M/E level.
Capricious appetite, rejects at sight or smell of food.
This general symptom is much more highly marked than the M/E symptom following.
Weak memory.
Very sensitive.
Again this is a vague symptom and of little use in prescribing as it stands. We may even place these last two behind the next symptom, which is a highly marked and individualized particular.
Stools jelly-like with blood and mucus.
In a live patient there should be no doubt as to the order of the hierarchy, but here in a paper case there is much room for interpretation.
The remaining particulars could be ordered as follows:
Colic better bending double.
This symptom refers to the function of the digestive system.
Joints painful, red and hot.
I have put this before hydrothorax because it has clearer modalities.
Hydrothorax.
This symptom simply describes the state of an organ. It tells us little.
Urine hot.
Here we have the product of disorder but little information about the disorder.
Stiff neck.
Now we know a little about this part but it is less serious than any of the above.

10) *Cannot bear anyone walking about in the room.*
This is the only M/E and is sufficiently unusual to be given first place in the hierarchy.
Feels paralysed and unable to move.
This very disturbing symptom might greatly restrict the patient. It may fall under the heading of 'delusions' and thus be M/E, or it may be a disturbance of the sensorium, CNS – either might refer to consciousness, which is a function of an organ, the brain.
Flushes of heat upwards.
This is a clear general symptom.
Pains in the joints move about at night ⎱ Both of these two particulars have
Hot dry throat worse eating sweet things ⎰ clear, striking modalities that are almost S,R&P.
Empty sensation in the abdomen.
This is a sensation in a major area of the anatomy.
Thick, rust-coloured sputum.
Although this is a product it is more descriptive than the next.
Red face with distended veins.

And this symptom says more than:
Tickling cough.
Note from the above that a symptom may change its place in the hierarchy according to
  its intensity
  its modalities
  its relevance to the disease process
  its timing – recent symptoms take precedence.
Thus any case must be analysed individually, and according to its own merits.

Lesson 5

REVISION – MORE HIERARCHIES

1) *She easily loses confidence, especially in new situations.*
M/E temperament.
Frightening dreams especially at night.
There may be a tendency to put this symptom before the last, and this could be justified because it is more intense, and has a clearer modality. However, I have put it second because in this case I feel it relates less to personality than to digestion!
Inclined to faint with menses.
This is a strong reaction to a metabolic process. One should check the patient's iron levels.
Menses protracted.
This is a metabolic process – a general.
Constipation plagues her.
This is an intense symptom of digestive malfunction, a general.
Blowing noises in the ear.
This is a distinctive particular, but nevertheless a particular.

2) *Likes to be alone.*
An M/E symptom.
Sinking feeling in the abdomen around mid-morning.
I have put this symptom in this position on the assumption that it is connected with appetite.
Otherwise it is relegated behind the next two symptoms.
Worse becoming heated } Both of these are generals, but I have favoured the first
Tendency to take cold } as a general modality.
Ulcers in the mouth } I have arranged these three particulars according to the
Dry mouth } degree to which they restrict the patient.
Dry skin }

3) *Worse since lost wife.*
This is the point at which the temperament changed, but note that more probing is essential to use this symptom in prescribing, e.g. is he grieved or lonely or what?
Pessimistic.
M/E describing personality.
Squeezing pain right temple, worse morning and worse moving.
This is a particular with a clear description and two modalities.
Scraping pain on the tibia worse at night.
This is a particular with a clear description and one modality. It may also represent a different stage in the disease process from the last symptom.

4) *Urine stops and starts, refusing to flow continuously.*
S,R&P. The significance of this symptom may drop according to how long the patient has had it, and also according to the intensity of the other symptoms, particularly the next.
Dizzy turning the head to either side.
This is a disturbance of consciousness. Perhaps it may be due to physical

disturbance such as arthritis in the cervical spine, in which case it may well be a common symptom.
Dullness of consciousness.
This is the state of the constitution. Often there are physical causes but it refers more specifically to the level of degeneration.
Sweats profusely at night.
This is a marked general symptom.
Constipation.
This is also a general symptom but less marked than the last.

5) *Pains wander from joint to joint.*
This is an unusual and individual state of the economy that could be described a S,R&P.
Worse wet is a modality of the above symptom.
Fear of thunderstorms.
This M/E symptom goes next.
Worse becoming cold.
This is a highly marked modality on the general level.
Worse after alcohol.
This is a general, but less highly marked than the above as it indicates an element of choice.

6) *Avoids company.*
This is an M/E.
Worse alcohol.
This is a general modality.
Thick yellow catarrh comes in strings.
Because this is a clearly described particular we put it before the next two symptoms, even though it is a product of disease.
Very foul breath.
I have put this in this position because of the implied intensity, otherwise it might go last.
Weight in the pit of the stomach after alcohol ⎫ Both of these are particulars but
Ulcers on the tongue ⎭ one has a modality.

7) *Coldness in spots.*
This is S,R&P.
Numbness as if something crawling over the skin.
This is also S,R&P. This one refers more to the skin as an organ, whereas the first is akin to a general.
Restless.
Although an M/E symptom, this is rather vague as it stands.
Worse change of the weather.
This is a general symptom.
Diarrhoea after eating fruit.
This is a little more peculiar than abdominal cramps on eating, so it comes first.
Abdominal cramps on eating.

8) *Worse since split up with boyfriend.*
This is clearly the exciting cause, but we must delve deeper to get the exact symptom, e.g. is it disappointed love, offence, anger suppressed, etc.?
Worse dwelling on unpleasant thoughts.
This is an M/E that describes the main mental state.
Worse sun ⎫ These are general modalities and it could be argued that
Worse before menses ⎭ 'worse before menses' could be ordered with first, as it describes an event that causes periodic change in the metabolism.
Thirst in the evening.
This is a general symptom of appetite, but unlike the next symptom it has a modality.
Desires salt.

Throbbing headache in the morning, worse before menses.
This is a particular symptom.

9) There are a lot of mentals in this case. To decide which goes first you must ask which restricts him most. You could argue to put any of these symptoms first, and once again I must be evasive and say it depends on the individual patient.
Anxious person who is easily excited.
This symptom may have the strongest impact on him.
Enthusiastic but easily discouraged.
This may describe the temperament.
Dislikes to be alone but shy of company.
Again this describes the temperament.
Difficult to concentrate on his studies.
There might be a temptation to put this first, especially if it is a recent symptom.
Polyps in the left ear is a particular symptom.

10) In this case we have a presenting symptom that greatly restricts the patient, yet our success in dealing with it will depend on how well we link it into the total symptom picture.
Easily angered and wants to beat up others because feels violent.
This is an M/E symptom.
Suspicious.
This may describe the personality and/or may be an underlying cause of the anger, in which case we would put it before the anger.
Worse before menses ⎫ Both of these are general modalities. There is an
Worse after sleep ⎬ inclination to put the second first because it is a daily
                  ⎭ occurrence after a natural process. I have put 'worse menses' first because of its rhythm.
Hiccoughs worse eating, worse drinking, worse talking.
This is a particular symptom with clear modalities, and therefore also a valuable prescribing symptom.
In this exercise I have used not the language of the Repertory but the language of the patient.
When you have covered the relevant lessons later on, you may find this exercise useful to repertorize and gain further experience of putting the patient's symptoms into the language of the Repertory, and also to gain experience of finding the remedy.

Lesson 6

ACTIVITY 4	The answer to the True or False are as follows:
	True
	True
	False
	False
	False
	True
	True
	True
	True
	True
	True
	True
	True
	True
	True
	False

	False
	False
	True
	True

Lesson 8

ACTIVITY 3

1) Check your answers with the text.
2) Check your answers with the text.
3)
a. 6th or 30th potency, depending on the patient's energy, severe physical reaction.
b. 30th potency; a 6th potency might be sufficient for the wound, but 30th will prevent any general reaction or tetanus.
c. IM potency, strong emotion.
d. 6th potency might be sufficient, or might need repetition later, physical.
e. 30th potency because of severity of the symptoms.
f. 30th potency, because a child is very sensitive; this is an acute unless you have other information (which you should look for anyway).
g. 6th potency and visit the dentist.
h. 6th potency, repeated as the pain recurs, physical and needs time to heal.
i. 30th potency because this is the exit to the lymph system and therefore possible systemic origin; check this out.
j. 30th potency because of severity of physical. The two concomitant symptoms suggest deeper reaction so look for it.
k. 30th or 200th potency depending on the energy of the patient, because this reaction is on the emotional level.
l. IM or 10M potency. This is a constitutional problem so needs to be moved deeply. You will need the rest of the TSP to prescribe.
m. 6th potency in a child, 30th in an adult, because a physical symptom with a definite exciting cause.
n. 30th or 200th potency depending on the energy of the patient, because this is a severe reaction although through the excretory organs.
o. 6th potency immediately will prevent any sequence because on the physical level and clear exciting cause.
p. 6th potency on occurrence because physical.
q. 6th or 30th potency, depending on the energy of the patient and the resistance of the complaint.
r. 200th to IM potency because constitutional and general condition affecting mental level.
s. 30th potency may be sufficient; 200th might be indicated because of the emotional reaction of the faint.
t. IM or 10M as this is a constitutional problem.

Lesson 11

ACTIVITY 8

Symptom	Page
Pain behind the ear, better in the open air	307
A crack down the middle of the tongue	399
Pustular eruptions on the abdomen	547
Pain in the region of the umbilicus	571
Palpitations at 3 a.m.	874
Hand itchy after rubbing	1022
Partial paralysis of the foot	1180
Patient worse from brandy consumption	1344

Symptom	Page
Sensation of fullness in the head	118
Pain in the eye as if from sand	258
Painless ulcers on the lower lip	428
Empty sensations in the stomach during nausea	489
Abdominal pain as if squeezed between two stones	560
Bowel movements olive green	638
Fear of pins	46
Sensitive to the slightest noise	79
Aversion to her own sex	95
Moist eruption on the head	116
Eyes dry on reading	238
Nose bleeding from the right side	335
Burning heat on the upper lip	385
Lower jaw twitches	395
Constant inclination to clench the teeth together	431
Discharge from the back of the nose	333
Nausea during headache	508
Cancer of the ovaries	715
Bloody discharge after menstruation	721
Sensation of a plug in the larynx	755
Racking cough at night	801
Sensation as if a weight on the chest	839
Swelling of the axillary glands	880
Pain in the back with desire to urinate	898
Cold hands during fever	959
Dark redness of the tonsils	450
Sleep disturbed by dreams	1235
Patient worse after taking butter	1362
Fatigue after eating	1370

ACTIVITY 10

Symptom	Page	Type of symptom
Numbness in the forearm in the morning	1303	Part
Pulsation deep in the inguinal region	1037	Part
Falling backwards during convulsions	599	General
Skin itches when walking in the open air	1353	Part and (?) S,R&P
Nausea on waking	509	General
Greedy for money and possessions	9	M/E
Mucus membrane of mouth discoloured blue	400	Part
Dizzy and nauseous	101	General
Feels rejected	49	M/E
Worse after eating pork	1363	General
Low back pain as if crushed	922	Part
Hawks up hard mucus plugs	816	Part
Worse after taking clothes off	1410	General (or ?S,R&P)
Wounds heal slowly	1422	General
Urine smells sweet	688	Part
Sensation of a lump rising in throat	750	Part
Jaws clenched	356	Part
Objects seem too large	280	Part
Unable to keep eyes open	247	Part
Cannot make up his mind about anything	57	M/E
Laughs constantly	61	M/E
The head feels empty when talking	115	S,R&P
Feels knotted inside	1370	Part
Wrings the hands and gesticulates	50	M/E
Lump in the left breast	838	Part

Stitching pain in the armpit	865	Part
Wakes before midnight	1255	General
Symptoms aggravated when sweating	1391	General
Everything feels unreal	91	M/E
No feelings or sensations on the skin	1330	Part

Glossary of Terms

Acute disease	In homoeopathy this term refers to a self-limiting episode or illness from which the patient either recovers or dies.
Aggravation	The initial increase in the intensity of symptoms when the activity of the vital force is increased, e.g. by a remedy.
Allopathy	The practice of treating disease by reversing the symptoms, usually by giving a medicine that creates the opposite effect of that produced by the body in reacting to disease.
Amelioration	A decrease in the intensity of symptoms which naturally follows the aggravation phase.
Ayurvedic medicine	The ancient medical system of India.
Causation	The exciting or maintaining causes that activate the inherent predispositions of an individual; the original morbific agent.
Chronic disease	In homoeopathy this term refers to a state of debility in which the vital force has been damaged in such a way that it cannot regain health.
Centesimal scale	The strength of the medicine is diluted 1:100.
Concomitant symptoms	A symptom that occurs at the same time as another symptom. There is seldom any relationship between the two, except in time.
Constitution	This term indicates that individuals can be classified according to the characteristic reaction pattern of the vital force, i.e. there are patterns of chronic illness.
Crude dose	A medicine which has not been potentized in any way.
Cure	The permanent removal of a patient's symptoms.
Decimal scale	The strength of the medicine is diluted 1:10.
Diagnosis	A term used by the allopath in labelling patterns of symptoms into the commonly occurring groups.
Dosage	In homoeopathy this term refers to the number of times a remedy is given.
Double-blind trial	This is a term used to describe drug trials when neither the patient nor the supervisor knows the nature of the drug, or even which patient has received the drug or the placebo until after all the data are collected.
Endemic disease	A term used when a group of symptoms is associated with a particular place or environment.
Epidemic disease	A term used when a group of symptoms is associated with a particular time or disturbance which is virulent enough in nature to affect a very large proportion of the population.
Exciting cause	A detrimental factor to which each individual is particularly sensitive, so the predisposition or weakness of the vital force is exposed.
Herb	Plant of medicinal value. The term is not used to refer to the potentized preparation from this plant. Herbalism is the use of medicinal plants to effect an improvement in health. These may be prepared in tincture or dried, etc., but they are not potentized and the practice does not usually involve the use of the basic homoeopathic laws such as the Law of Similars, the single remedy, the single dose or the Law of Cure.
Hierarchy of symptoms	See page 25 of the text.

Holistic	When the patient is treated in such a way that each symptom is related to the whole.
Homoeopathy	The practice of treating disease by administration of a medicine capable of producing the very same symptoms.
Idiosyncrasy	An individual's peculiar sensitivities.
Isopathy	The practice of treating disease with the self-same agent that caused the patterns of symptoms.
Keynote	A particularly characteristic symptom that identifies a remedy.
Maintaining cause	A detrimental factor inimical to life which lowers the vitality of an individual, thus making him or her more susceptible to ill health.
Materia Medica	A delineation of the possible action of a remedy; a list of symptoms the remedy may produce and cure; a collection of symptom pictures of homoeopathic remedies.
Miasm	A chronic affliction of the vital force from which it cannot recover.
Minimum dose	That amount required to stimulate the vital force to react.
Modality	That which affects change to a symptom.
Morbific agent	That which is capable of disturbing the activity of a vital force.
Natural medicine	A substance which is unprocessed or changed in any way; a process whereby the body's own reactions are enhanced, as these are recognized as the quickest and safest way to cure.
Naturopathy	A process of cure using the natural reaction of the body to disease.
Objective symptoms	One that is observable through the senses.
Orthodox/western medicine	That commonly accepted in Europe, North America, Oceania, etc., as established practice based on allopathic procedures and an extensive search for objective data.
Palliation	When the symptoms are ameliorated without cure.
Placebo	When the patient believes he or she has taken a medicine when in fact the 'pill' was unmedicated.
Point of change	The point at which a pattern of symptoms originates.
Potency	The number of times a homoeopathic medicine has been diluted and succussed.
Potentization	The process of diluting and succussing to prepare a homoeopathic remedy.
Predisposition	The inherent weaknesses in the vital force which arise from miasms.
Prescribing symptoms	An unusual or distinctive symptom that characterizes the patient or his or her illness.
Presenting symptoms	Those symptoms of which the patient first complains and brings to the practitioner to receive help.
Prognosis	A forecast or prediction as to how the pattern of symptoms will change.
Prover	A person who takes a homoeopathic remedy with the intention of proving it.
Proving	When a homoeopathic medicine is taken by a healthy person to discover what symptoms it is capable of producing.
Pseudochronic disease	Originates from a maintaining cause, and as such will disappear when the cause is removed.
Quinnism	The original name given to homoeopathy when it first came to Britain.
Remedy	The name given to a homoeopathic medicine; it is never called a drug.

Repertory	A dictionary of the symptoms produced by homoeopathic remedies.
Resonance	Vibrating in unison with.
Similimum	The remedy that can produce a symptom picture most similar to that of a patient.
Sporadic disease	A disease which selects individuals at scattered distances and times.
Subjective symptom	One that is experienced only by the patient.
Succussion	The process of vigorously shaking a solution of the medicine during its preparation and between dilutions.
Suppression	When the symptoms disappear, but not according to the Law of Cure.
Susceptibility	The degree of sensitivity to the remedy or to the exciting cause.
Symptom	An awareness of discomfort or dis-ease which is abnormal to the patient.
Symptom picture	May be applied to the patient or to a remedy. It is the characteristic group of symptoms produced by either of these.
Tincture	A medical substance prepared in alcohol.
Total symptom picture	Contains the *entire* symptom picture of the patient.
Vital force	The process or intelligence that corrects and maintains the organism within a set pattern.
Vitalism	A system of medicine that recognizes that the organism is more than a collection of chemicals. It recognizes the principle of life.
Vitality	The amount of energy available to sustain life.

Bibliography

P   Blackie M 1981 The challenge of homoeopathy. Unwin, London

Borland D 1982 Homoeopathy in practice. Beaconsfield, London

Bott V 1978 Introduction to anthroposophical medicine. Rudolph Steiner Press, London

*   Campbell A 1984 Two faces of homoeopathy. Jain, New Delhi

*   Capra F 1983 The turning point. Collins, London

Capra F 1975 The tao of physics. Shambala, London

*   Close S 1985 The genius of homoeopathy. Jain, New Delhi

P   Coulter H 1980 Homoeopathic science and modern medicine. North Atlantic Books, Berkeley, USA

*   Coulter H 1973 The divided legacy. North Atlantic Books, Berkeley, USA

*   Dubois R 1965 Man adapting. Yale University Press, New Haven

A   Dudgeon R E 1978 Lectures in the theory and practice of homoeopathy. Jain, New Delhi

Grahamann G 1974 The plant. Rudolph Steiner Press, London

Hahnemann S 1971 The organon. Jain, New Delhi

Hauschka R 1983 The nature of substance. Rudolph Steiner Press, London

*   Henry C 1983 Analytical repertory of the symptoms of the mind. Jain, New Delhi

Hume Douglas E 1989 Pasteur exposed. Bookreal, Australia

*   Illich I 1977 Medical nemesis. Penguin, London

*   Leonard G 1981 The silent pulse. Wild Woodhouse, London

*   Kent J T 1970 Lectures on homoeopathic philosophy. Jain, New Delhi

A   Kent J T 1985 Lesser writing. Jain, New Delhi

Kent J T 1986 The repertory. Jain, New Delhi

Mees L F C 1984 The secrets of the skeleton. Rudolph Steiner Press, New York

Miller R J Comparative value symptoms in the selection of the remedy. Jain, New Delhi

Mills S 1988 Alternatives in healing. MacMillan, London

Nash E B How to take a case. Jain, New Delhi

Neatby E A, Stonham T G 1987 A manual of homoeopathic therapeutics. Foxlee-Vaughan, London

*   Phatak S R 1963 A concise repertory of homoeopathic medicines. Homoeopathic Medical Pub, Bombay

*   Rakat H A 1985 Boenninghausen's therapeutic pocket book. Jain, New Delhi

P   Riley A, Cunningham P J 1979 The fake pocket medical dictionary. Faber & Faber, London

Roberts H 1988 The principles and art of cure of homoeopathy. Jain, New Delhi

Roberts H 1937 Sensations as if . . . . Boericke & Tafel Inc

Schmidt P 1976 The art of interrogation. Homoeopathic Medical Pub, Bombay

Schmidt P 1976 The art of case taking. Homoeopathic Medical Pub, Bombay

*   Schwenk T 1965 Sensitive chaos. Rudolph Steiner Press, London

*   Shepherd D 1953 Homoeopathy for the first aider. Health Science Press, London

P   Shepherd D 1964 Magic of the minimum dose. Health Science Press, London

*   Shepherd D 1967 Homoeopathy in epidemic diseases. Health Science Press, London

P   Shepherd D 1974 More magic of the minimum dose. Health Science Press, London

Shepherd D A physicians posy. Health Science Press, London

Speight P 1979 A course in homoeopathy. Health Science Press, London

*   Tyler M Different ways of finding the remedy. World homoeopathic, New Delhi

Ullman D 1989 Medicine of the twentieth century. Thorsons, London

*   Von Boenninghausen C 1979 A systematic alphabetical repertory of homoeopathy. Jain, New Delhi

A   Von Boenninghausen C 1979 Lesser writings. Jain, New Delhi

P   Vithoulkas G P 1979 Homoeopathy and the new man. Thorsons, London

*   Vithoulkas G P 1980 The science of homoeopathy. Thorsons, London

     Weir J The art and science of homoeopathy, Jain, New Delhi

*   Whitmont E C 1980 Psyche and substance. North Atlantic Books, Berkeley, USA

     Wright H 1977 A study course in homoeopathy. Furmor, St Louis, USA

*   Recommended

P   Good precourse reading

A   Advanced work

Index